BEAT THE BOARDS!

(I Just Did)

Melissa Umphlett, MD
Pathology Resident
Washington Hospital Center
Washington, DC

THE ULTIMATE GUIDE TO ACE STEP 2 OF THE USMLE

JONES AND BARTLETT PUBLISHERS

Sudbury, Massachusetts

BOSTON   TORONTO   LONDON   SINGAPORE

World Headquarters
Jones and Bartlett Publishers
40 Tall Pine Drive
Sudbury, MA 01776
978-443-5000
info@jbpub.com
www.jbpub.com

Jones and Bartlett Publishers Canada
6339 Ormindale Way
Mississauga, Ontario L5V 1J2
CANADA

Jones and Bartlett Publishers International
Barb House, Barb Mews
London W6 7PA
UK

Jones and Bartlett's books and products are available through most bookstores and online booksellers. To contact Jones and Bartlett Publishers directly, call 800-832-0034, fax 978-443-8000, or visit our website, www.jbpub.com.

Substantial discounts on bulk quantities of Jones and Bartlett's publications are available to corporations, professional associations, and other qualified organizations. For details and specific discount information, contact the special sales department at Jones and Bartlett via the above contact information or send an email to specialsales@jbpub.com.

Library of Congress Cataloging-in-Publication Data

Umphlett, Melissa.
   Beat the boards! (I just did) : the ultimate guide to ace step 2 of the
USMLE / Melissa Umphlett.
     p. ; cm.
   Includes index.
   ISBN-13: 978-0-7637-4123-5
   ISBN-10: 0-7637-4123-X
   1. Medicine—Outlines, syllabi, etc. 2. Medicine—Examinations,
questions, etc. 3. Physicians—Licenses—United States—Examinations
—Study guides.   I. Title.
   [DNLM: 1. Medicine, Clinical—Examination Questions.   WB 18.2
U52b 2007]
   R834.5.U47 2007
   610.76--dc22
                                        2006021179
6048

Production Credits
Executive Publisher: Christopher Davis
Associate Editor: Kathy Richardson
Associate Production Editor: Alison Meier
Associate Marketing Manager: Laura Kavigian
Manufacturing Buyer: Therese Connell
Interior Design and Composition: Shawn Girsberger
Cover Design: Timothy Dziewit
Cover Images: © Jones and Bartlett Publishers. Photographed by Kimberly Potvin.
Printing and Binding: D. B. Hess
Cover Printing: D. B. Hess

Printed in the United States of America
10 09 08 07 06   10 9 8 7 6 5 4 3 2 1

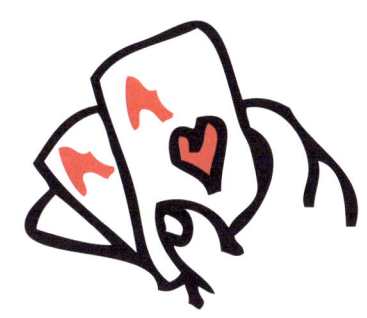

I dedicate this book to the VIDD

who were my inspiration.

CONTENTS

SECTION 2 CLINICAL SKILLS. 241

x

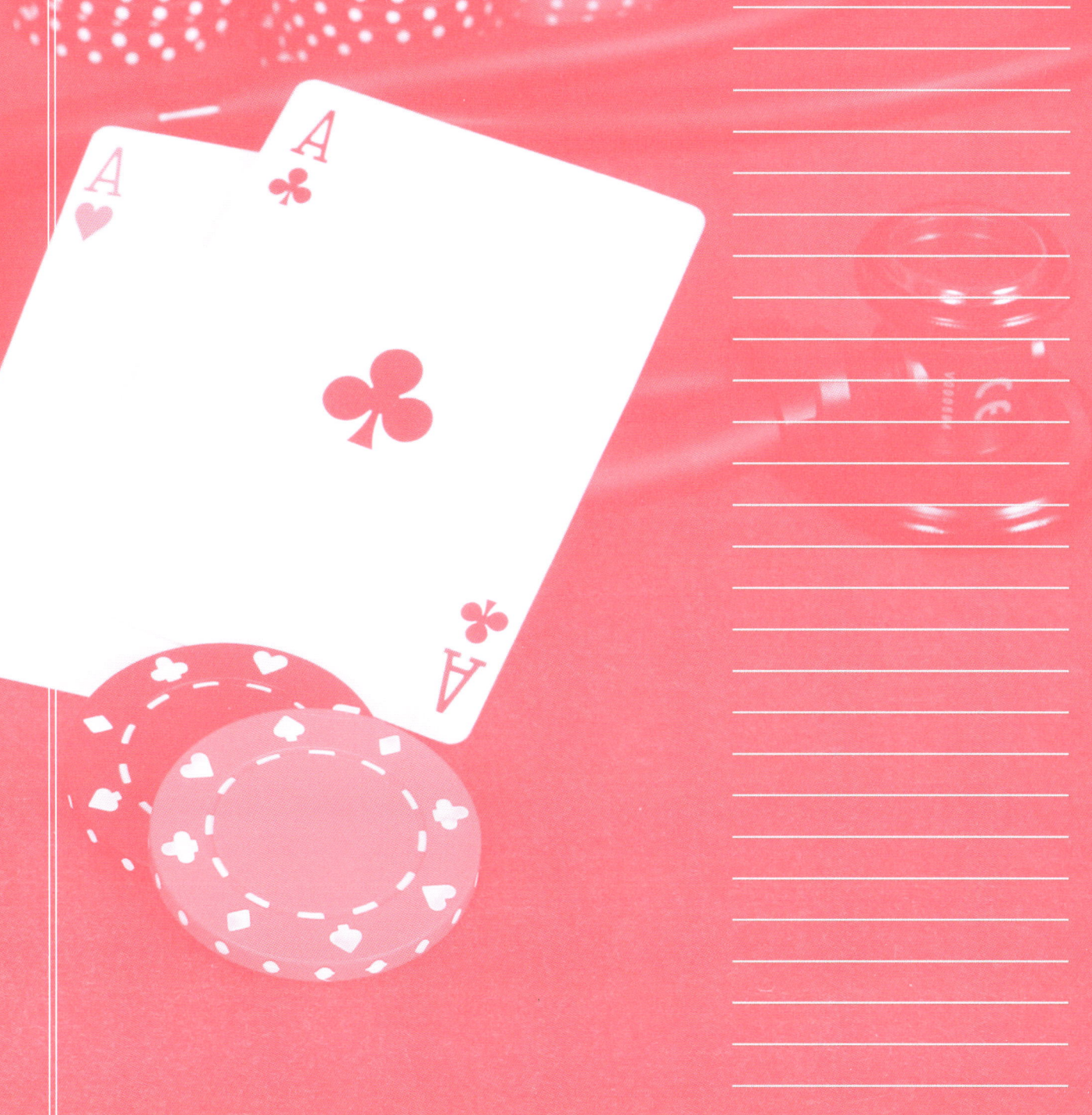

SECTION 1

CLINICAL KNOWLEDGE

CHAPTER 1 GETTING STARTED

This book is designed to serve as a complete review for USMLE Step 2 CK and CS. I am sure you recognize the importance of getting a good score on your boards. Obtaining a good score carries a large weight in the residency match program. Your score can make or break your chance of getting the residency you desire. I am providing a book that will prepare you for both parts of Step 2, a book full of insider material because I just took the exam.

I wrote this book because I am full of knowledge as a result of my recent exam, and I want to share this knowledge with you. While my friends and I were studying for the exam, I was exposed to almost every major review book on the market today, including bootleg copies from highly marketed courses. I felt that these review books were incomplete in many areas and excessive in others. I understand that most students are crunched for study time. Around Step 2 time, everyone is trying to complete rotations, prepare for the residency match, and study. It is imperative not only to study hard, but also to study smart. That is what this book will do for you. I spent much of my study time reading review books, answering tons of review questions, figuring out the test format, and formulating strategy. In this time I figured out quite a bit about this exam and how to achieve the score you want on it. As we all know, the correct answer may not be true to your personal experience in the hospital; the correct answer is what the National Board of Medical Examiners wants to hear.

Step 2 has gone through a radical change in recent years, and other review books have not caught up with the revisions. The passing score has been raised to 182, and many students find it just as difficult as Step 1. The important thing to remember is *don't underestimate this test*! If you speak with people who took Step 2 two years ago, many of them will say that it is easy, you only need to study for two weeks, and you should do a few review questions. That is not true anymore.

You don't have to take an expensive review course with volumes of required reading. I have compiled all the test-worthy information with no fluff. All you need to do is study like a madman with the time you have and follow my recommendations about practice questions. Trust me, you will rock the test; I know because I just did.

INSIDER STUDY TIPS

I have designed this book to appeal to all different kinds of learning styles. At this point in the game I am sure that you know how you personally study effectively. Some people are text learners; some people learn better by illustrations and visualization. I have attempted to incorporate different modes of learning to appeal to all types of students. I know sitting for hours is not great fun; I have just tried to make your hours spent as effective as possible.

I highly recommend taking some time off to study if you can spare it. I took Step 2 CK after studying for a little more than six weeks while in a "light rotation." I completed around 2500 review questions in that time. I highly recommend a subscription to usmleworld.com; this Web site has the absolute best review questions on the market. I can honestly say they are indicative of what you will see on the actual exam. The question length, content, wording, and answer choices are very similar to what is actually on the test. The site's question bank is the best and is less expensive than others on the market. Also, if you decide to move your test date to make more time to study, usmleworld.com gives you the option of extending your subscription for a week or two for a reduced rate instead of paying for another month. Don't let your score discourage you when you begin these questions. Read the disclaimer on the Web site and keep in mind that a score of 50–60% is OK! Keep up the good work; your score will improve. Don't be discouraged; these questions are excellent, and the explanations are awesome. Once you have been practicing these questions for a week or two, try a few questions from other sites, and they will seem easy to you. That is because they *are* too easy and have not caught up with Step 2 as it is now. I will provide a more in-depth discussion of CS study methods when we reach Section 2: Clinical Skills, but I also recommend usmleworld.com's practice cases. They are more than sufficient and cover almost all of the possibilities you will see on the test.

STUDY STRATEGIES

Once you sign up for the test, make a study schedule and stick to it. The best thing I can tell you to do is set aside the proper amount of time for each discipline in the test. I recommend the following.

Based on a Six-Week Study Period
- OB/GYN: 1 week
- Peds: 1 week (or maybe 5–6 days)
- Surgery: 1 week
- Internal Medicine: 1 week

During the last two weeks, review all the information again and increase the number of practice questions you complete.

Make room for ethics, epidemiology, biostatistics, and psychiatry in this time. This is just a guideline. Only you know what you are weakest in and what you need to spend more time on. Follow your instincts and your averages on the practice questions.

This schedule may seem strange because of the length of time I recommend for OB/GYN and pediatrics, but *do it*. You will be amazed at the number of questions on these two topics. They should be considered just as important as surgery and internal medicine. I know it sounds crazy, but it is true. Also, I know how it is: If you are not considering peds or OB/GYN as a specialty, or if it has simply been a while since you have had these rotations, you really forget the material. It's not material you use much in other rotations, and it gets pushed to the back of your mind. Honestly, what medical student can rattle off rare enzyme deficiency disorders and genetic diseases on a given day without a little preparation? That information is practically designed to fly out of your mind a few days after you review it.

I can't stress this fact enough: Just because you may not be particularly interested in these subjects, the NBME is. And the whole point of preparing for the exam is to play the game and get every possible answer correct.

Surgery questions may be presented a little differently than you would expect. Besides the basic surgery we all have learned, the exam presents *many* emergency trauma questions. Also, basic principles will get you a long way.

Internal medicine is the broadest topic on the exam. What I mean by this is that there is a lot of information within the discipline of internal medicine. Just remember, there are not actually more questions on the exam about internal medicine, but knowledge of internal medicine principles is needed to correctly answer many of the questions.

Easy Points That You Should Not Miss

Psychiatry questions on the exam are straightforward; you can dedicate less time to this discipline, but *do not* ignore it. These should be easy points to add to your score. The goal is to make sure you get the easy questions right.

Ethics and epidemiology questions also offer easy points. Just read the material and you're golden. Actually, I recommend writing down common biostatistics formulas on a handy sheet of paper and reading it a day or two before the exam, and the morning of your exam on the train ride, bus ride, or drive. As soon as you get in the testing center, write down the formulas on the sheets provided; that way they are there and you won't miss easy points on the exam.

In each section of the book I will point out many topics that will be heavily tested on the exam.

LOGICAL ADVICE FOR TAKING THE EXAM

When thinking about possible questions you will encounter on your personal exam, remember the reason for the exam. Passing this exam is one of the major milestones before you are awarded a medical license. *The NBME is trying to test whether or not you are ready to be a doctor, someone who knows what to do for a patient in life-threatening situations.* When you are reviewing, pay special attention to what I like to call "your patient could die any second" cases. For example, I can guarantee you will see questions involving meningococcal meningitis, MI, difficult delivery situations, pneumothorax, PE, and trauma. Therefore, when you are studying, KNOW these topics.

What You Really Need to Know

You Must Know:

1. How to recognize the disease
2. Every possible step en route to diagnosis
3. Treatment

Another high yield point is to know the diagnostic criteria for all major diseases.

Memorize cutoff lab values. "What would you do next?" is the most popular question on the exam.

Know for Each Disease:

1. All tests to be ordered (in order)
2. "Gold standard" or diagnostic test
3. Least expensive test (when applicable)

Many people feel that questions on Step 2 tend to be vague. The point is to see the answer that the NBME wants.

Clinicals are an excellent learning experience. The knowledge you gain will stay in your mind much more than any material you can learn from a book.

I will provide logarithms for steps to proper diagnosis. In addition, I have included Quick Tip, Here's the Deal, and Pay Attention! features that will point out the right answer for you in black and white. Learn them! I know that the procedure presented in the correct answer is not always practical, but it is what the NBME considers to be the right answer. For example, who uses a V/Q scan to detect a PE anymore? Is the CT machine broken? Just remember you want to get the question correct, so give them what they want.

CAUTION: What you may have done in your hospital may not be the right answer on the test.

Testing Strategy

Practice makes perfect. Do the practice questions and pay attention to what they are asking. Read the explanations to your incorrect answers and figure out where you went wrong. What in the question was misleading to you? Did you miss an important detail? Learn from the explanation so you don't make that mistake on the test. I printed out the explanations to my wrong answers and carried them around with me in the weeks before the exam. When I had free time I would look them over (on the subway, etc.). It may sound like walking around with a "scarlet letter" on your chest, but it worked.

If your study plan is six weeks, by the fifth week you should have a good handle on the material, working through any weak points and continuing to complete plenty of practice questions. In the last two weeks, increase the number of questions you are doing each day. Remember, this test is longer that Step 1. You need to train for the long day of concentrating. Trust me, during your final block you don't want to blow it off or lose focus. When going for a competitive score, every question counts. If you were going to run a marathon, would you only run two miles a day while training for the race? You can train the stamina of your mind. When completing your practice questions, do blocks of 46. Try completing two or three consecutive blocks instead of taking breaks in between each block. Use what works for you.

The Real Test

Total number of questions: 400.

9 blocks containing 46 questions.

Total time: 9 hours.

Skip the tutorial; this will give you extra time.

Use the testing strategy that works for you (breaks vs no breaks).

Eat light on test day; don't divert blood flow away from your brain to your GI tract with a big meal.

Don't let other people at the testing center freak you out. You know the people I am referring to: the panicky, strung out, flight-of-ideas person who is taking Step 1 for the first time. Another good example is the overconfident student taking the exam who claims that it is sooooo easy. Don't let these people distract you; bring an MP3 player and make yourself less accessible.

The testing center is usually cold, so bring a sweatshirt or something comfortable to wear.

Answering Questions and Time Strategy During Blocks

Practice the methods previously discussed when you are completing your practice questions. These methods really work, but they require a little practice to feel confident using them.

When reading the test question, read the first sentence, and then read the last sentence. The first sentence usually will give you the patient's presenting complaint/ situation and age. The last sentence asks the question; for example, what do you do next? What is the best initial diagnostic test? Or what is the best treatment?

Reading each question in this manner shows you what to look for in the body of the question stem. Many times you will find that you don't need to read all of the information in the question stem to derive the correct answer. Many of the questions will be almost half a page long and will include a list of lab values that keeps you scrolling to even reach the answer choices. You will find that most of that information is extraneous.

For example, I encountered questions that presented a patient with age and chief complaint in the first sentence. After reading that sentence you will know right away what the diagnosis is. Half a page of vitals, extraneous information, and many lab values followed this information. The last sentence asked, what is this disease commonly associated with? This is an answer you can come up with easily without reading the entire question. Save that time to answer the more challenging questions that require more thought.

During the test you should use your time to answer as many questions correctly as possible. If the question seems confusing and you cannot narrow the answer choices to two, mark the question and move on. Don't spend five minutes on a question you obviously don't know. At the end of the block use the extra time to look at the difficult question again, after you have conquered all of the easier questions in the block.

Many of the questions will have 10 or more answer choices. Decide what you think the answer is before you look at the choices. Many of the choices will be similar, and this can easily make you question whether or not you are thinking of the right answer. Remember, your first answer *is* best. If you have studied this book and completed the review questions don't second-guess yourself, because you don't need to!

On the actual exam, the answer choices will appear in alphabetical order. So stick to your first answer, quickly find it alphabetically, and move on.

MY HOPES FOR YOU

While reading this book, I want you to feel like you are reading the notes of an encouraging friend who wrote down everything she remembered from the test for you. Other review books are written by people who took the exam more than 10 years ago or, even better, 5 people who took the exam more than 10 years ago. Step 1 may remain relatively unchanged, but Step 2 has made some BIG changes that are *not* reflected in the competitors' texts.

I spent numerous hours preparing this book to contain everything you need to know, without any filler. You now have everything you need to know, so relax. Honestly, I hope that you love this book. Now, go ace the test and tell all of your friends to buy this book!

CHAPTER 2 BIOSTATISTICS

This section is a low-yield section, so do not spend too much time on it. When I took the test, I wrote down the formulas and the following chart as soon as the test started (see Figure 2-1) and remembered this information:

Sensitivity = A/(A + C)
Specificity = D/(B + D)
PPV = A/(A + B)
NPV = D/(D + C)
Odds Ratio = (A x D)/(B x D)
Relative Risk = [A/(A + B)] / [C/(C + D)]
Attributable Risk = [A/(A + B)] – [C/(C + D)]

FIGURE 2-1 Cheat Sheet

Disease

		+	−
Test	**+**	A	B
	−	C	D

BIOSTATISTICS

Incidence: Number of new cases of a disease per unit of time.

Prevalence: Total number of cases of disease (new or old) at a particular time.

Reliability (precision): Measures the reproducibility and consistency of a test.

Validity (accuracy): Measures whether or not the test measures what it claims to measure.

Relative Risk (RR): Disease risk in exposed population vs unexposed population. Only used after experimental or prospective study.

RR > 1 — significant

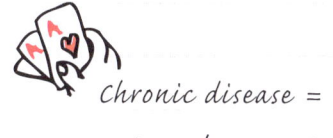

Chronic disease =
Prevalence > Incidence
Acute illness =
Incidence < Prevalence

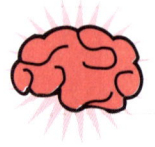

sensitivity rules OUT.

Specificity rules IN.

Ideally, a test should be

sensitive and specific.

PPV and NPV are affected

by disease prevalence.

If cutoff value for a disease is

raised = more false negatives

and fewer false positives.

If cutoff value for a disease is

lowered = fewer false negatives

and more false positives.

Odds Ratio (OR): Disease in exposed and no disease in unexposed with no disease in exposed and disease in unexposed. Less accurate way to calculate RR.

Attributable Risk (AR): Comparison of incidence rate of a disease in exposed vs unexposed patients. Number of cases associated with one risk factor. Used in prospective/cohort studies.

Sensitivity: Probability that a diseased patient will test positive for the disease.

> Sensitive test = Good screening test. Many false positives, but it doesn't miss many people with the disease.

> (1 − sensitivity) = false negative ratio

Specificity: Probability that a healthy person will test negative for the disease.

> Specific tests = Disease confirmation; they do not call anyone sick who is actually healthy.

> (1 − specificity) = false positive ratio

PPV: Probability of having a disease given a positive test result.

> Higher Prevalence = Higher PPV

> Highly Sensitive Test = Higher False Positive = Lower PPV

NPV: Probability of not having a disease given a negative test result.

> Higher Prevalence = Lower NPV

> Highly Sensitive Test + Higher False Positive = Higher NPV

Correlation Coefficient: Degree of relationship between two variables. Range is −1 to +1.

> 0: No association.

> +1: When one variable increases, the other variable increases.

> −1: When one variable increases, the other variable decreases (inversely).

Confidence Interval (CI): The mean value of a data set usually does not equal the real mean of a population. CI = 95% implies there is a 95% chance that the population mean will fall within a certain range.

DATA COMPARISON

t-Test: Compares two means.
Analysis of Variance (ANOVA): Compares three or more means.
Chi-Square Test: Used to compare nonnumeric data (percentages).
Meta-analysis: A compilation of statistical data from many studies (see Figure 2-2).

FIGURE 2-2 Bell-Shaped or Normal Distribution.

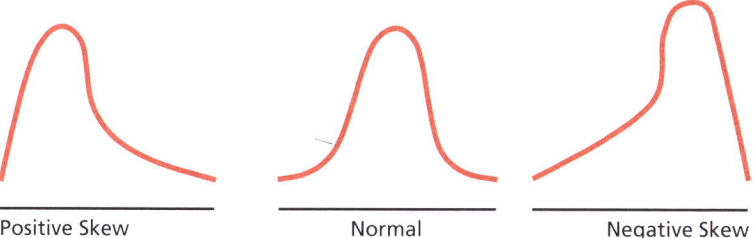

Positive Skew   Normal   Negative Skew

.

Mean: Average.
Median: Middle number (if in a list the number that would be in the middle of the list).
Mode: Most common number.
  In a normal distribution Mean > Median > Mode.
Skewed Distribution: Not a normal distribution.
Positive Skew: Tail on right; Mean > Median > Mode (lots of higher values).
Negative Skew: Tail on left; Mean < Median < Mode (lots of lower values).
_p_-value: < 0.05 means there is a 5% chance the data were obtained by chance or random error.
  $p < 0.05$ is commonly the cutoff value in medical studies. No matter what the p-value is, a study can still have flaws and not have clinical significance.
Null Hypothesis: Hypothesis that states the results were obtained by chance or error.
  $p < 0.05$ means there is a 5% chance the null hypothesis is correct..
  In studies you hope to reject the null hypothesis..
Type I Error: Rejecting the null hypothesis when it is true (making unfounded claims).
Type II Error: Accepting the null hypothesis when it is false.
Power: Chance that a study will reject the null hypothesis when it is indeed false.

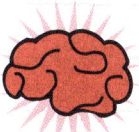

Three means ANOVA has three syllables.

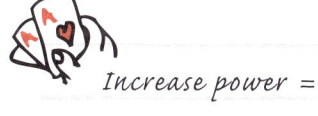

Standard Deviation (SD)
1 SD = has 68% of values
2 SD = has 95% of values
3 SD = has 99.7% of values

Increase power =
Increase sample size

BIAS

Confounding Variable: Unmeasured variable that affects the independent and dependent variable; may lead to false conclusions about the study.

Enrollment Bias: Study groups are not equal as a result of not randomly assigning the subjects.

Nonresponse Bias: People fail to respond to the surveys.

Lead-Time Bias: Bias due to time difference (study shows prolonged survival, but perceived prolonged survival is actually because screening advances the survival time).

Recall Bias: When subject over- or underestimates risk factors; this is a risk in retrospective study.

Interviewer Bias: A result of failing to blind the person administering the study.

Unacceptability Bias: When patients in the study want to please the study administrator and therefore do not report their behavior accurately.

COMMON STUDIES

Experimental: One variable is manipulated, and its effects are studied in two equal patient groups.

Prevalence/Cross-Sectional Survey: Prevalence of disease vs prevalence of risk factors; best tested using prospective study.

Retrospective/Case-Control Study: Subjects with disease (cases) and subjects without disease (control) are chosen.

Cohort Study: Divide a sample population into two groups based on presence or absence of a risk factor; follow the groups over time and watch for disease development.

CHAPTER 3 CARDIOLOGY

There will be some ECGs on the exam. Enough information is provided in the question stem to pick the correct answer without spending time interpreting the ECG. Therefore, if you are not the best at reading ECGs don't bother learning every rare ECG change for this exam. For a review of heart sounds and ECG, see Figure 3-1. Fortunately, the cardiology questions on the exam are on common problems you should recognize. Relax! Type A personality is associated with cardiovascular disease, and we don't want that.

FIGURE 3-1 Heart Sounds and ECG

P: depolarization of atria
PR: AV node
QRS: depolarization of ventricles
Q–T: ventricular contraction
T: repolarization of ventricle

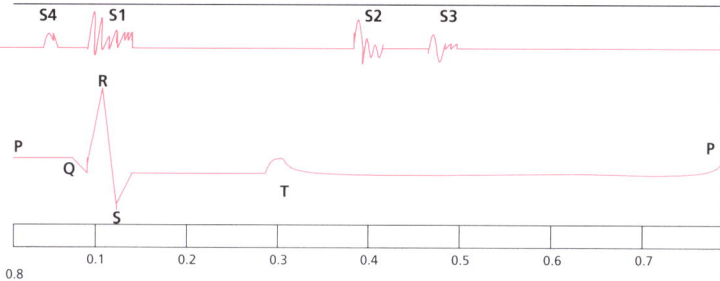

REVIEW OF HEART SOUNDS AND ECG

Normal Heart Sounds
S1: Mitral and tricuspid closure
S2: Aortic and pulmonary closure

Abnormal Heart Sounds
S3: Dilation
S4: Hypertrophy

For congenital heart defects, see Chapter 14, "Pediatrics."

There are a few cardiology-related equations you should memorize. They are provided in Table 3-1.

TABLE 3-1 Helpful Equations

Cardiac Output = Heart Rate × Stroke Volume	CO = HR × SV
Ejection Fraction = $\dfrac{\text{Stroke Volume}}{\text{End Diastolic Volume}} \times 100\%$	EF = SV/EDV × 100%
Mean Arterial Pressure = Cardiac Output × Total Peripheral Resistance	MAP = CO × TPR
Systolic – Diastolic = Stroke Volume	S – D = SV
Stroke Volume = Pulse Pressure	SV = PP

CARDIAC MURMURS

Mitral Regurgitation: Soft S1 Associated with mitral valve prolapse	Radiates to axilla
Mitral Prolapse: Midsystolic click Associated with panic disorder	Commonly in young women
Mitral Stenosis: Loud S1 Associated with rheumatic fever	Opening snap
Aortic Regurgitation: Audible S3 LV dilatation	Widened pulse pressure
Aortic Stenosis: S3/S4 ejection click Harsh systolic ejection murmur Possibly caused by bicuspid valve problem	Radiates to carotid

AV HEART BLOCK

Arrhythmias
Sinus Bradycardia: Vent rate < 60 bpm.
>   Normal in athletes.
>   If needed treat with atropine; see Table 3-2.

TABLE 3-2 Sinus Bradycardia

First degree	PR interval > 0.2
(Mobitz I) Second degree Wenckebach	Increased PR followed by drop beat Drugs can cause this
(Mobitz II) Second degree	Drop beat but no change in PR Conduction problem is cause Can progress to third degree
(Complete) Third degree	P and QRS have no relation Atrial and ventrical miscommunication

Sinus Tachycardia: Vent rate > 100 bpm
  Caused by normal autonomic response to exercise, fear, stress
PSVT: Normal QRS rate 150–250 bpm
  Caused by AV node reentry
Atrial Flutter: Atrial rate 300 bpm; P wave saw tooth
  Anticoagulation
  TEE—check for clot in atrium
Atrial Fibrillation: Wavy; no P waves
  Anticoagulation, rate control, Ca+ channel, B-blocker, digoxin
  TEE—check for clot in atrium
Premature Ventricular Contractions: No P followed by wide early QRS
  Lidocaine if needed
Ventricular Tachycardia: Widened QRS + 3 or more consecutive PVCs
  Lidocaine
Ventricular Fibrillation: Tracing completely irregular
  Immediate shock

Right Branch Bundle Block and Left Branch Bundle Block

RBBB: QRS duration > 0.12 sec; may be a sign of lung disease	**LBBB:** Possible heart disease sign; possible sign of cardiovascular disease

WOLFF PARKINSON-WHITE SYNDROME

Cause: Alternate electrical pathway between atria and ventricle
Presentation: Palpitations
ECG: Short PR and delta waves
Treatment: Quinidine or procainamide; do not give digoxin or verapamil
Surgery: Radiofrequency catheter ablation

ANGINA

Crushing substernal chest pain lasting around 20 minutes.

Three Types of Angina

STABLE ANGINA
- Pain on exertion; stress remits with rest.
- Pain *is* relieved by nitroglycerin.
- ECG: ST depression with pain or normal ECG with no pain.
- Pain lasts less than 20 minutes.
- **Treatment:** Nitroglycerin.

UNSTABLE ANGINA
- Prolonged chest pain that begins with rest.
- Pain is *not* relieved by nitroglycerin.
- ECG: ST depression with pain.
- Defined as change in frequency or intensity of stable angina episodes.
- Cardiac enzymes are normal.
- **Treatment:** IV heparin; PTCA if pain does not resolve.

VARIANT (PRINZMETAL'S) ANGINA
- Chest pain at rest.
- Pain is *not* relieved by nitroglycerin.
- ECG: ST elevation at rest.
- Cardiac enzymes are normal.
- Caused by coronary artery spasm.
- **Long-term treatment:** Ca+ channel blockers (diltiazam).

MYOCARDIAL INFARCTION

Presentation: Crushing substernal chest pain with or without radiation to jaw, arm, and shoulder.
   Not reproducible by palpation.
   Lasts longer than 30 minutes.
   Pain is *not* relieved with nitroglycerin.
   New murmur, distended neck veins, hypotension.

Diagnostic Tests: Echo to look for ventricular wall abnormality; most specific blood test for MI is Trop 1; X-ray to look for cardiomegaly or pulmonary congestion.
   See Table 3-3 for myocardial infarction markers.

Chronological ECG changes: Peaked T waves, ST elevation, T wave inversion, Q waves.

Anterior Wall Infarct: Increased risk for arterial thrombosis.

FIGURE 3-2 ECG Changes in an Inferior Wall Infarct

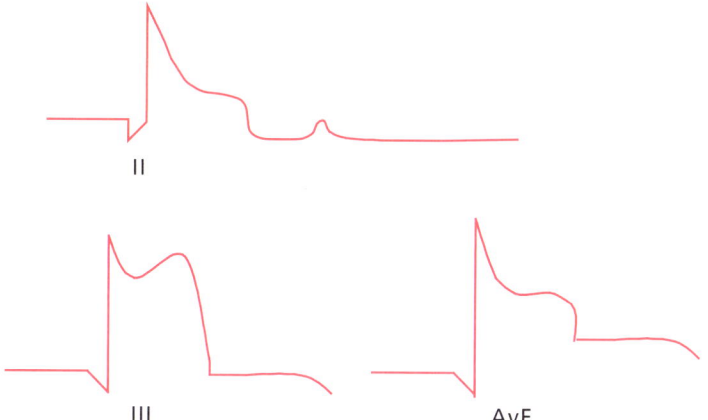

TABLE 3-3 Myocardial Infarction Markers

LDH 1	Found primarily in myocardium Rises at 24 hours Peaks at 48 hours Positive for 72 hours (Day 1, 2, 3)
CKMB	Best for the first 24 hours Rises at 6 hours Peaks at 12 hours Positive for 24 hours
Troponin 1	Most specific test Rises at 2 hours Peaks at 2 days Positive for 7 days

Complications

Dressler's Syndrome: (1–2 weeks post MI) autoimmune reaction; pericarditis, pleural effusion, fever, increased ESR and leukocytes

Treatment: "**MAIN BOAT**" plus ECG monitoring (don't give B-blocker if DM)

Morphine	**B**-blocker—decreases incidence of second MI
MI **A**CE **I**nhibitor— if EF < 40%	**O**$_2$
Nitroglycerin	**A**SA
	tPA & Heparin

V Tach: Treat with lidocaine; see Figure 3-3.
Ejection Fraction: Best predictor of survival.
Lethal Arrhythmia: Most common cause of death post-MI.

FIGURE 3-3 V Tach

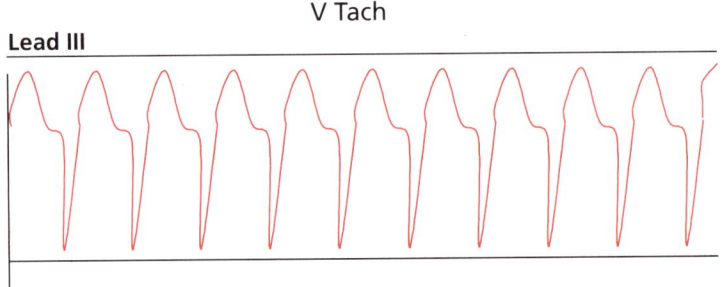

V Tach

Lead III

OTHER CAUSES OF CHEST PAIN

Pleuritis
Seen with pneumonia.

Pericarditis
Inflamed pericardial sac with or without cardial effusion. Cough, fever, chest pain when *lying down.*

Causes: MC—after viral URI (Coxsackie), uremia, drugs, autoimmune, malignancy

Diagnostic Tests: Friction rub, ST segment elevation, increased ESR

Treatment: NSAIDs, ASA, or steroids; pericardiocentesis if necessary

Cardiac Tamponade
Decreased cardiac output; common cause is stab wound.
Diagnostic Tests: CXR, ECG
Treatment: Pericardiocentesis

Costochondritis
More common in women and reproducible on palpation.
Self-limited.

Esophageal Problems
Achalasia, spasm, nutcracker.
Must rule out MI with these disease processes.

GERD
Heartburn; worse when lying down.
Cause: LES relaxation; commonly seen with hiatal hernias
and increased intra-abdominal pressure

Idiopathic Hypertrophic Subaortic Stenosis
AD in about half the cases.
Ventricular and intraventricular septum hypertrophy, which
decreases filling; see Figure 3-4.
An increase in cardiac contractility; or if blood volume falls
low, this will cause filling to decrease even more, which
will cause sudden death.
Presentation: Usually asymptomatic, but patient may
experience syncope
Diagnostic Test: S4, systolic ejection murmur; murmur more
prominent with Valsalva; murmur less prominent with
hand grip
ECG: Q waves, LVH
Confirmatory Test: Echocardiogram reveals LV wall
hypertrophy and outflow obstruction
Treatment: B-blocker

IHSS is the most common cause of unexpected death in young and healthy patients.

"Teen athlete drops dead during a game" = IHSS

FIGURE 3-4 IHSS

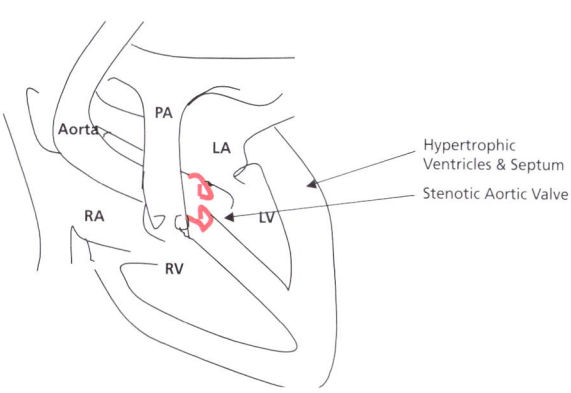

Aorta
PA
LA
RA
LV
RV

Hypertrophic
Ventricles & Septum
Stenotic Aortic Valve

Restrictive Cardiomyopathy

Contractile and filling dysfunction from scarring and fibrosis.

Causes: Drugs, sarcoid, hemochromatosis, amyloid, radiation, fibroelastosis

Diagnostic Test: Abnormal biopsy

Treatment: Lower fluid load (no cure known)

Constrictive Pericarditis

Thickened pericardium.

Key: "Knock" heard on exam—this determines if restrictive vs constrictive pericarditis

Diagnostic Test: Normal ventricular biopsy

Treatment: Remove pericardium (curative)

Primary Dilated Cardiomyopathy

Systolic dysfunction and LV dilation.

Causes: Chagas, cocaine, doxirubicin, beriberi, alcohol abuse, myocarditis

Presentation: Audible S3

Diagnostic Test: CXR; balloon heart ECG changes

Confirmatory Test: Echocardiography

Treatment: Diuretics, ACE, B-blockers; implantable cardiac defibrillator if EF < 35

Congestive Heart Failure

Systolic ejection dysfunction, leading to inappropriate oxygenation of tissues.

High Mortality: People who suffer from MI are more likely to die from CHF.

Risk Factors: CAD, HTN, heart disease, renal failure, anemia

Presentation: Orthopnea (sleeps with many pillows due to discomfort in breathing when lying down); PND; JVD (right heart failure); S3 and S4, hepatomegaly/ascites (right heart failure); pulmonary edema—CHF at its worst

Diagnostic Tests: Transthoracic echo to assess EF; CXR— cardiomegaly (LVF and RVF); Kerley B Lines, pulmonary congestion (LVF)

Initial Treatment: (good for pulmonary edema) ACE inhibitor—greatly decreases mortality; inotrope, diuretics, morphine (causes pulmonary venous constriction)

Stable CHF Treatment: Na+ restriction, B-blocker, ACE

NEW YORK HEART ASSOCIATION CHF FUNCTIONAL CLASSIFICATION

- Class 1: No activity limitation; no symptoms with normal activity
- Class 2: Slight activity limitation; comfortable at rest and mild exertion
- Class 3: Marked activity limitation; comfortable *only* at rest
- Class 4: Symptoms present at rest; discomfort with any physical activity; confined to bed or chair

Cor Pulmonale

Right ventricular enlargement due to lung disease (idiopathic, COPD, pulmonary embolism)

Presentation: Cyanosis, clubbing, loud P2, right-sided S4, tachypnea
Treatment: Management with Ca+ channel blockers
Cure: Heart/lung transplant

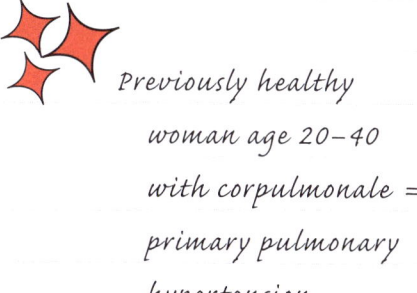

Previously healthy woman age 20–40 with corpulmonale = primary pulmonary hypertension.

Hypertension

Screening every 2 years starting at age 3.

3 measurements on 3 separate occasions of > 140/90 mmHg separated by 2 weeks in time; see Table 3-4 for blood pressure classification.

Exceptions to 3 separate measurements rule:

1. Pregnancy
2. Severe HTN > 210 systolic; > 120 diastolic
3. Evidence of end organ damage

HTN in pregnancy is discussed in Chapter 13, "Obstetrics."

TABLE 3-4 BP Classification

BP Classification (Normal < 130/85)	
Normal (High) Checkup 1 year	130–139/85–89
Stage I: Confirm within 2 months	140–159/90–99
Stage II: Evaluate/care within 1 month	160–179/100–119
Stage III: Evaluate/care within 1 week	180–209/110–119
Stage IV: Immediate emergency	> 210/120

Hypertensive Emergency

BP > 200/120 mmHg (end organ damage)

Hypertensive Urgency

BP > 200/120 mmHg (no end organ damage)

Don't wait for 3 BP measurements.

Elevation of systolic or diastolic alone is still considered hypertension.

Most common cause of death in untreated HTN patients?

Coronary artery disease

Best way to prevent stroke:

HTN control

Diagnostic Tests: Assess risk factors, cause, organ health, ECG, lab tests—urinalysis, chem. 7 H and H.

Treatment Goal: Maintain BP >140/95.

Try to keep BP even lower in diabetics and renal disease patients.

See Table 3-5 for HTN treatment.

TABLE 3-5 HTN Treatment

Antihypertensive Treatments	Effective for:
Diet and exercise	Beneficial for everyone!
Ca+ Ch blockers	Peripheral vascular disease, migraines, Raynaud's, claudication, Prinzmetal's angina
Diuretics	African Americans and osteoporosis, CHF
B-blockers	CAD, migraines, isolated systolic HTN, MI (decreases reoccurrence)
ACE inhibitors	DM (renal protective) Side effect—cough

End Organ Damage S&S: MI; dizzy, blurred vision (on fundoscopic exam—copper wire nicking or AV nicking); HA, papilledema, and left ventricular dysfunction from having to pump blood against so much pressure

URGENT/EMERGENCY HTN TREATMENT
- Nitroprusside (decreases preload and afterload because it is a veno- and arterial dilator).
- B-blocker.
- Nitroglycerin—venodilator only; contraindicated in patient who is currently on sildenafil. Both drugs together cause severe hypotension, so in emergency situations always inquire!

PRIMARY ESSENTIAL HTN (IDIOPATHIC)
Most common cause of HTN (> 90% of cases)
Risk factors: Age, smoking, obesity, family history, high Na+, diet

SECONDARY HYPERTENSION
Identifiable causes of HTN

Causes:

- **Coarctation of the Aorta:** Seen in children and in patients with Turner's Syndrome, in half the body only.
- **Fibrous Dysplasia of Renal Vasculature:** Bruit plus HTN; test: IVP; can be corrected with angioplasty.
- **Young Woman:** Oral contraceptive pills (very common).
- **Young Man:** Sometimes seen with excessive alcohol intake.
- **Conn's Syndrome:** Caused by aldosterone-secreting tumor; HTN, hypokalemia, metabolic alkalosis, and low renin.
- **Pheochromocytoma:** HTN that comes and goes, urinary catecholamines.
- **Cushing Syndrome**
- **Elderly:** Atherosclerosis causes renovascular HTN; new onset HTN and renal bruit in older patient.

CORONARY ARTERY DISEASE

Coronary Artery Disease Risk Factors

- Hypercholesterolemia: high triglycerides alone are not a risk factor.
- Hypertension: diagnosed by proper guidelines.
- Smoking.
- DM: obesity is not a risk factor.
- Low HDL: < 35 mg/dl.
- Age: ≥ 45 in men; ≥ 55 in women (or women in menopause with no estrogen replacement—estrogen increases HDL).
- Family history of premature CHD in first-degree relative.
- History of MI in father less than 55 years old or mother less than 65 years old.

See Table 3-6 for cholesterol screening and treatment guidelines.

TABLE 3-6 Cholesterol Screening and Treatment

No Risk Factors	2+ Risk Factors	Treatment
Total Cholesterol > 239 HDL < 35	Total Cholesterol > 200 HDL < 35	Measure fasting LPL
LDL < 160	LDL < 130	Remeasure in 1 year
LDL 160–189	LDL 130–159	Diet
LDL > 189	LDL > 159	Meds

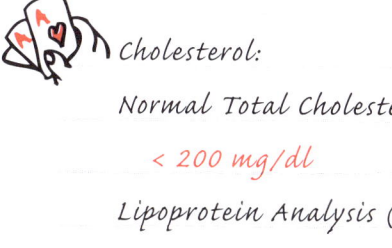

Incidence of CAD increases with high cholesterol. CAD may manifest as: MI, CHF, angina.

Measure total cholesterol and HDL every 5 years starting at 20 years old.

Cholesterol:
Normal Total Cholesterol:
< 200 mg/dl
Lipoprotein Analysis (LPL):
Total Cholesterol − HDL − (Triglycerides/5) = LDL

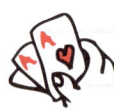

HDL: The "Good Cholesterol"

Protective against
*   atherosclerosis*
HDL increased by:
exercise, estrogen, 1–2
*   alcoholic drinks per day*
*   (not 10 on Saturday*
*   night)*
HDL decreased by:
smoking, progesterone,
*   elevated triglycerides*

Surgical manipulation
*   of arterial tree causes*
*   increased risk for*
*   cholesterol embolism.*

Secondary Causes of Hyperlipidemia

Secondary causes of hyperlipidemia could be steroids, B-blockers, OCPs, uremia, nephritic syndrome, and alcoholism.

Familial Hypercholesterolemia

Corneal arcus, xanthelasmas (fat pads on tendons), and xanthomas (fat pads on eyelids).

Pancreatitis with *no risk factors* is pathognomonic for familial hypercholesterolemia.

Treatment: Allow 3–6 months to modify diet and begin exercise plan before beginning drug therapy.

Statins: HMG CoA reductase inhibitors are excellent at lowering cholesterol because they stop its production; most effective when taken around 8:00 p.m. (side effects—myositis, liver function impairment).

Niacin: Still first-line treatment but not tolerated well (side effect—intense pruritis).

Cholestyramine: Bile acid sequestration (side effect—gas).

Gemfibrozil: Lipoprotein lipase inhibitors (no longer commonly prescribed).

VASCULAR DISEASE

Vascular disease is also covered in Chapter 19, "Surgery."

Abdominal Aortic Aneurysm (AAA)

Most common cause is atherosclerosis.

Presentation: Asymptomatic, or the classic presentation is pulsatile mass in abdomen.

Diagnostic Test: Verify size with U/S or CT scan.

Treatment: 6 cm > elective surgery; less than 4 cm, check in 2 years; tender on palpation, immediate surgery (can be fatal).

Dissecting aneurysm has "ripping pain in abdomen radiating to back.".

May have associated peripheral artery aneurysm.

Aortoiliac Disease

Butt claudication and impotence

Intermittent Claudication

Exacerbated by exercise

Alleviated by rest

Associated symptoms of decreased blood flow (decreased temp, weak pulse, cyanosis)

Diagnosis: Doppler (if pressure gradient is present, order arteriogram).

Treatment: *Must* quit smoking.

B-blockers are contraindicated.

If disease interferes with work or lifestyle, treat with revascularization.

CHAPTER 4 DERMATOLOGY

ACNE VULGARIS

Propionibacterium acnes is an anaerobic bacteria that lives in the bottom of pores. If the pilosebaceous glands get clogged, this provides the anaerobic background for P. acnes to flourish and multiply. This is how the open comedones or whiteheads are formed.

Unrelated to diet.

Common in adolescents; men are not affected after growing subsides because it is directly related to hormones that affect sebaceous gland production.

Women can be afflicted with adult onset acne due to the same mechanism that affects boys in adolescence.

Treatment:

> First—Topical benzoyl peroxide; topical clindamycin.
> Second—Oral tetracycline or erythromycin and topical tretinoins.
> Last Resort—Isotretinoin (oral) vitamin A analogue that is highly teratogenic; pregnancy test (negative) and BCP compliance are required for prescription; side effects include night blindness, severe dry skin and mucosa, muscle pain, and elevated LFTs.

ECZEMA (ATOPIC DERMATITIS)

Family and personal history of asthma, allergies.

Begins in childhood, chronic, usually worse in winter.

Pruritis, dry scaling, reddish areas (head, upper extremities).

Excess itching can lead to breach in skin and increased risk of infection.

Associated with elevated IgE (also associated with asthma and allergy).

Diagnostic Tests: Clinical diagnosis

Treatment: Topical steroids, emollients

PSORIASIS (T-CELL MEDIATED)

Well-demarcated salmon plaques with white scales.

On head, knees, and elbows.

Nails appear broken and lifting from nail bed.

No pruritis.

Diagnostic Tests: Biopsy—Munro abscesses, with neutrophils

Sometimes associated with arthritis and lithium

Treatment: UV light therapy, steroids

ACANTHOSIS NIGRICANS

Dark areas associated with malignancy, drugs, diabetes.
Sometimes described by patient as "dirty-looking."
Investigate underlying cause (always carefully rule out
malignancy).

BULLOUS PEMPHIGOID

Large itchy bullae in patients more than 60 years old.
Negative Nikolsky's sign.
No mucous membrane involvement.
Pruritis present.
Dermal–epidermal junction involvement.
Diagnostic Tests: Neutrophils at dermal–epidermal junction
Treatment: Steroids

PEMPHIGUS VULGARIS

Blisters on skin and mucous membranes in patients less
than 60 years old.
Positive Nikolsky's sign (pressure = lateral blister extension).
Mucosa membrane involvement.
Pruritis absent.
Intradermal involvement.
Associated weight loss, malaise, autoimmune.
Diagnostic Tests: Intradermal bullae immunoflourescense
IgG and C3 deposits
Treatment: Steroids

CELLULITIS

Fever plus all signs of infection in affected area (swollen,
tender, red).
Deep subcutaneous tissue involvement.
Commonly associated with coexisting condition that causes
a fissure or break in the skin.
Most Common Causes: First—group A strep; second—staph
Treatment: Oral antibiotics; if immunocompromised, IV
antibiotics

LICHEN PLANUS

Oral mucosal lesions plus itchy *purple* polygonal-shaped
lesions.

Associated with Hepatitis C!
Diagnostic Test: Hyperkeratosis upon biopsy
Treatment: Steroids

LICHEN SCLEROSIS

Atrophic plaques on genital region with dilated sweat glands.
Affects middle-aged women.
Key Presentation: Middle-aged woman notices change in genital skin
Diagnostic Test: Biopsy—keratin-plugged sweat ducts, collagen bands, and atrophy

IMPETIGO

Itchy honey-crusted lesions.
Causes: Coag positive staph—if furuncle is present (bullous type)
Strep—if no furuncle with or without glomerulonephritis (nonbullous type)
Treatment: Antibiotics

Contagious! Don't share clothes or towels.

ROSACEA

Red papules on face that are sometimes confused with acne; exacerbated by heat, sun, alcohol.
Begins in middle age.
Classic Presentation: 50-year-old with big nose and symmetric red, flushed face
Treatment: Tetracycline; severe/refractory—isotretinoin

SEBORRHEIC DERMATITIS

Scaling skin on head and eyelids, "halo."
Treatment: Dandruff shampoo

ACTINIC KERATOSIS

Red patch with white scales.
Related to sun exposure.
Can lead to squamous cell CA.

ERYTHEMA NODOSUM

Tender, red spots, usually on shins.
Look for coexisting disease (usually autoimmune).

ERYTHEMA MULTIFORME

Target lesions, even on palms and soles.
Seen after some infections (mono, herpes) and drugs (listed in Stevens-Johnson syndrome).
Treatment: Stop the cause.

TOXIC EPIDERMAL LYSIS SYNDROME/ STEVENS-JOHNSON SYNDROME

Drug reaction (1–3 weeks after new drug ingestion).
Key Presentation: Target lesions on face, mouth, and conjunctiva
Involves mucous membrane positive Nikolsky's sign; epidermis becomes necrotic
Associated drugs that cause reaction:

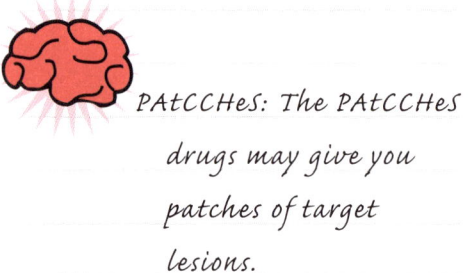

PAtCCHes: The PAtCCHes drugs may give you patches of target lesions.

Phenylbutazone
Allopurinol
Cephalosporins
Carbamazepine
Hydantoin
Sulfas

Treatment: Discontinue drug, prescribe steroids and fluids.
(Mild form is erythema multiforme [target lesions].)

SEBORRHEIC KERATOSIS

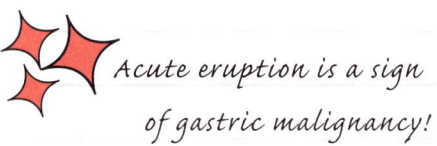

Acute eruption is a sign of gastric malignancy!

Looks like a large mole with a wartlike layer on top.
Treatment: Look for cancer; otherwise self-limited.

VARICELLA

Group of vesicles found along a dermatome (trunk, face).
Itchy lesions that progress to vesicles.
Passed via lesion contact or respiratory droplets.
Highly contagious! Infectivity begins around 1 day before eruption.

SHINGLES (VARICELLA ZOSTER)

Recurrent eruptions; associated with pain.
Treatment: Acyclovir.
Vaccine available.

VITILIGO

Skin depigmentation.
Often associated with antibodies to parietal cells.

LICE (PEDICULOSIS CAPITIS)

Common in grade school, spreads easily, and is extremely itchy.
Diagnostic Tests: Clinical; visualize on hair shaft.
Treatment: Premethrin cream; wash and high heat dry or sterilize all sheets, towels, clothing, brushes.
The former treatment lindane is neurotoxic and therefore no longer used.

CRABS (PEDICULOSIS PUBIS)

Same symptoms as above except itch in different area.
Sexually transmitted.

SCABIES (SARCOPTES SCABIEI)

Itchy mite burrows on fingers and flexor areas.
Commonly seen in college dormitories.
Diagnostic Tests: Scrape lesions and visualize microscopy.
Treatment: Same as lice/crabs.

FUNGAL INFECTION

Caused by microsporum (pets are reservoir) or trychophyton.
Tinea capitis: Scalp—swollen weepy scalp, with possible hair loss; head usually illuminates with Wood's lamp.
Tinea corporis: Ringworm—raised, red ring lesions with normal center, usually on trunk.
Tinea cruris: Jock itch.
Tinea pedia: Athlete's foot—itchy, dry web space of foot.
Tinea unguium: Onychomycosis—thick nail that looks as if something is beneath it.

Diagnostic Test: Scraping and KOH prep.
Treatment: Azoles.

PITYRIASIS VERSICOLOR (MALASSEZIA FURFUR)

Small, scaling, discolored areas on body (darker or lighter).
Key: Affected areas do not tan.
Diagnostic Tests: Scrape and use KOH or Wood's light.
Treatment: Shampoo containing selenium sulfide.

BALDING

Causes:

Alopecia areata—associated with antimicrosomal antibodies
Chemotherapy
Male pattern baldness—androgens
Trichotillomania—pulling out hair due to nervous condition or psychosis

CONTACT DERMATITIS

Red, extremely itchy rash of vesicles.
Occurs after exposure to cheap jewelry, poison ivy/oak, makeup, soap, detergents.
Type IV hypersensitivity reaction.
Treatment: Steroids, antihistamines, oatmeal prep.

DERMATITIS HERPETIFORMIS

Vesicles on anterior thigh in celiac sprue—gluten sensitivity.

URTICARIA

Pruritic, wheal and flair.

KELOID

Overgrowth of scar tissue; not seen in Caucasians.

KERATOCANTHOMA

Same appearance as squamous cell cancer.
Super-fast-growing facial lesion with crater.
Resolves spontaneously.
Diagnostic Test: Biopsy to differentiate from cancer.
Treatment: Watch closely! Keratocanthoma can turn into squamous cell cancer.

Keratocanthoma can be precancerous!

SKIN CANCER

All skin cancer is associated with sun exposure. Lesion description or biopsy results will lead you to the type of skin CA immediately. Basal cell and squamous cell are both slow-growing lesions, but if you get a question describing an old farmer with a lesion on his head who hasn't been to the doctor in 20 years, it's basal cell.

Always biopsy!

Counsel all patients to wear sunscreen.

Basal Cell Cancer
Most common skin cancer and is associated with sun exposure.
Presentation: Red-brownish papule/telangiectasias with white-clear small scales on and around the lesion.
Diagnostic Test: Biopsy—basophilic palisading cells.
Treatment: Surgical excision; basal cell typically grows deep. Never METS.

Squamous Cell Cancer
Red, crusty, usually small in diameter (oozy/crusty appearance).
Associated with actinic keratosis and sun.
Diagnostic Test: Biopsy—anaplastic cells
Treatment: Surgical excision
Almost never METS.

Melanoma = Most Deadly Cancer

Melanoma
Associated with family history and fair-skinned individuals.
Always investigate any lesion patient feels has changed!
Prognosis based on depth or thickness.
Diagnostic Test: Biopsy—atypical melanocytes
Treatment: Surgery, or surgery and chemo (if positive nodes are present or suspect METS)

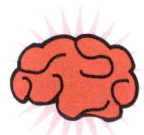

ABCD rule:

Asymmetric—shape of lesion

Border—that has become irregular

Color—any color change

Diameter—increase in size

CHAPTER 5 ELECTROLYTES

HYPERNATREMIA

Na+ > 145 mEq/L
Mental status changes, seizures, hyperreflexia

HYPONATREMIA

Na+ < 135 mEq/L
Mental status changes, seizures, cramps

HYPONATREMIA HYPERVOLEMIC

Rales, edema, JVD
Causes: CHF, nephrotic syndrome, cirrhosis, ADH

HYPONATREMIA HYPOVOLEMIC

Orthostasis, dry mucous membrane, decreased skin turgor
Causes: Fluid loss—diuretics, skin/GI/urine loss, sweating,
   burns
Treatment: H_2O to lower Na+

HYPONATREMIA NORMOVOLEMIC

Causes: Addison's disease, SIADH, psychogenic polydipsia,
   hypothyroidism
Diagnostic for SIADH: 2 x serum osm + 10 = urine osm
Treatment:
   Mild—fluid restriction
   Moderate (presence of neuro symptoms)—saline plus
      diuretics
   Severe—3% hypertonic saline plus some diuretics
   Chronic problem—demeclocycline

HYPERKALEMIA

K+ > 5 mEq/L
Common Causes: Crush injury/tissue destruction, renal
   failure, meds, adrenal insufficiency, acidosis
ECG—Tall peaked T waves, loss of P waves, wide QRS,
   prolonged PR interval
No ECG changes or symptoms with high K+: Hemolyzed
   sample! False high K+.

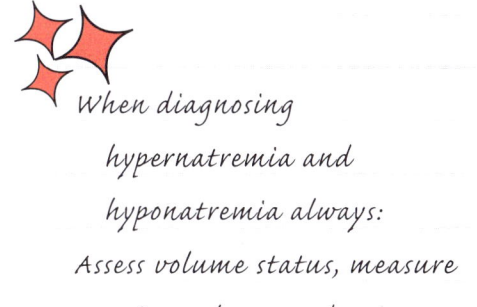

*When diagnosing
   hypernatremia and
   hyponatremia always:
Assess volume status, measure
   urine volume and urine osm.*

*Complications of changing
   Na+ level too rapidly*

- *1–2 mEq/L/Hr*
- *Too rapid drop:
   cerebral edema*
- *Too rapid rise:
   CPM (central pontine
   myelinolysis)*

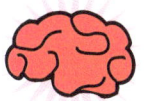

Treatment: "C BIG K"
Ca+ gluconate
   (cardioprotective)
Bicarbonate or **I**nsulin +
   Glucose
Kayexalate + loop diuretics

Alkalosis causes hypokalemia.

Acidosis causes hyperkalemia.

HYPOKALEMIA

K < 3.5 mEq/L
Muscle weakness, respiratory failure, cardiac arrhythmias
Common Causes: Insulin administration can cause low K+.
Treatment: Digitalis plus diuretics
ECG—Presence of U waves, flattening of T waves

HYPERCALCEMIA

Ca > 10.2 mg/dL
Usually asymptomatic
Severe—bones, stones, moans, psychiatric overtones
Common Cause: Hyperparathyroidism plus malignancy
ECG—QT interval shortening
Sometimes related to vitamin A derangement
Treatment: IV fluids, furosemide (thiazides are
    contraindicated), calcitonin, biphosphate (pamidronate),
    steroids

HYPOCALCEMIA

Ca < 8.5 mg/dL
Tetany, cramps, perioral tingling (Chvostek's sign and
    Trousseau's sign)
Common Causes: Hypoparathyroidism, renal insufficiency,
    vitamin D deficiency
ECG shows QT interval prolongation
Treatment: Ca+

HYPERMAGNESEMIA

Seen in pregnant patients being treated with Mg sulfate
Decreased DTRs, respiratory depression, hypotension, or
    patients with renal failure

HYPOMAGNESEMIA

Mg < 1.5 mEq/L
Usually seen in alcoholics (makes hypokalemia and
    hypocalcemia difficult to correct)

FIGURE 5-1 Acid/Base

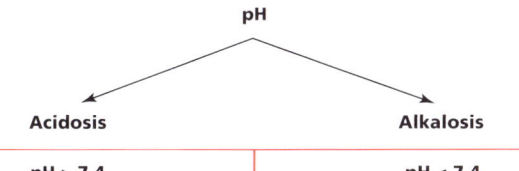

Acid/Base

pH	7.35–7.45
PO₂	75–105 mmHg
PCO₂	33–44 mmHg
HCO₃	22–28 mEq/L

pH

Acidosis   **Alkalosis**

pH > 7.4	**pH < 7.4**
High PCO₂ Respiratory Acidosis	**High PCO₂** Metabolic Alkalosis Compensation
Low PCO₂ Metabolic Acidosis Compensation	**Low PCO₂** Respiratory Alkalosis
High HCO₃ Respiratory Acidosis Compensation	**High HCO₃** Metabolic Alkalosis
Low HCO₃ Metabolic Acidosis	**Low HCO₃** Respiratory Alkalosis Compensation
Anion Gap	

Acidosis	**Alkalosis**
Respiratory: Elevated CO₂	**Respiratory:** Decreased CO₂
Obstructive Lung Disease: COPD	— (Initially) salicylate overdose—
— **B**ronchiectasis, **a**sthma, chronic **b**ronchitis, **e**mphysema	Alkalinize urine to speed excretion
— CNS depressants—barbiturates, benzos	**Keys:** Tinnitus, hyperventilation
Metabolic: Decreased HCO₃—MUDPILES	**Metabolic:** Elevated HCO₃—vomiting, diuretics, milk-alkali syndrome

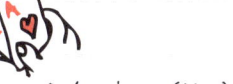

Potassium (K+) and Hydrogen (H+)

Elevated H+ = Elevated K+

Decreased H+ = Decreased K+

Example: Aldosterone Deficiency
= Metabolic Acidosis

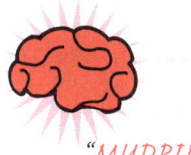

"MUDPILES"

Methanol
Uremia
Diabetic ketoacidosis
Paraldehyde ingestion
Ischemia, INH, iron
Lactic acidosis
Ethanol
Salicylates, starving

ANION GAP

Anion gap means there is a significant derangement of Na, HCO, or Cl. "MUDPILES" cause a decrease in HCO₃, which causes metabolic anion gap acidosis.

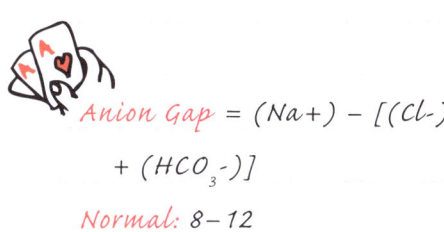

Anion Gap = (Na+) − [(Cl-)
+ (HCO₃-)]

Normal: 8–12

> 12: Metabolic Anion Gap
Acidosis

CHAPTER 6 ENDOCRINE

Endocrine disorders can be classified as primary or secondary (see Figure 6-1).

FIGURE 6-1 Primary vs Secondary Disorders

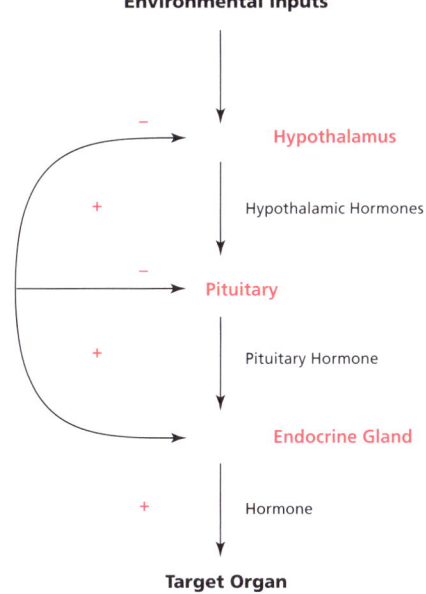

PRIMARY ENDOCRINE DYSFUNCTION

The endocrine gland itself is malfunctioning; the pituitary and hypothalamus are normal.
Example: Hyper- and hypothyroidism are usually primary.

SECONDARY ENDOCRINE DYSFUNCTION

The endocrine gland is normal, but the pituitary and hypothalamus are malfunctioning.

PITUITARY GLAND DISORDERS

Acromegaly
Pituitary growth hormone adenoma (benign)
Presentation: Coarse facial features; large jaws, feet, and hands; bitemporal hemianopsia; new onset diabetes
Diagnostic Tests: MRI reveals sellar lesion; do not rely on growth hormone levels!
Treatment: Surgical resection or ablation of tumor

Disorders Related to Growth Hormone
See Table 6-1 for a listing of growth hormone disorders.

In children, excess growth hormone is gigantism.

TABLE 6-1 Growth Hormone Disorders

Pygmies	Decreased growth hormone receptors; increased plasma growth hormone
Laron Dwarfism	Decreased tyrosine kinase receptors in limbs Normal growth hormone (Formerly known as midgets)
Dwarfs	Decreased sensitivity and amount of growth hormone

THYROID GLAND DISORDERS

Consider hypothyroidism in patients with unexplained increased CK and myopathy.

Hypothyroidism
Caused by low levels of thyroid hormone.
Presentation: Cold intolerance, fatigue, constipation, depression, and hoarseness
Diagnostic Tests: Increased TSH; decreased T3 and T4; low radioactive iodine uptake

CAUSES

Antiperoxidase is the most prevalent Ab in Hashimoto's.

Hashimoto's Thyroiditis
Associated with other autoimmune disease.
Presentation: Symmetric, nontender, nontoxic goiter
Key Diagnostic Labs: Antiperoxidase Ab, antimicrosomal Ab, and lymphocyte infiltration of the gland
Treatment: Levothyroxine

Subacute Thyroiditis
History of URI or mumps.
Key: Acute viral illness with fever and enlarged, tender thyroid gland
Treatment: Self-limited

Hashimoto's and subacute thyroiditis may cause transient hyperthyroidism before hypothyroidism.

Sick-Euthyroid Syndrome
May be caused by any illness.
Key: Decreased T3/T4 with normal TSH
Treatment: Self-limited

COMPLICATIONS

Myxedema Coma

Untreated severe hypothyroidism with mucopolysaccharide deposition in dermis and myocardium.

Trigger: Infection

Presentation: Hypothermia, hypoglycemia, shock, hypoventilation

Treatment: IV levothyroxine and IV hydrocortisone

Cretinism

Cognitive defects and physical abnormalities attributed to untreated congenital hypothyroidism.

Hyperthyroidism

Caused by high levels of T4.

Presentation: Heat intolerance, weight loss, nervousness, increased bowel frequency, tachycardia, tremor

CAUSES

Grave's Disease

Most common cause and primarily seen in women 20–40 years old

Key: Exophthalmos and pretibial myxedema unique to Grave's disease.

Diagnostic Tests: Thyroid stimulating immunoglobulins/thyroid stimulating Ab

Key: *Whole gland takes up excess radioactive iodine.*

Treatment:

> Mild—Methimazole, PTU
> Moderate—Radioactive thyroid ablation
> Pregnant patients—Thyroidectomy

Complications: Thyroid storm that causes high output cardiac failure with 25% mortality

Toxic Multinodular Goiter

Lumpy goiter without positive Abs.

Diagnostic Tests: Radioactive iodine uptake is high in the nodule but decreased in the rest of the gland.

Thyroid Nodules

Most thyroid nodules are benign, and the incidence increases with age.

Most common cause of thyroid nodule—hyperplastic colloid nodule.

Pregnant patients may have elevated TBGs, but free thyroid hormone and TSH are normal. Do not treat!

Most common cause of thyroid malignancy—papillary CA.
Diagnostic Tests: Whenever a patient presents with a thyroid nodule, measure TSH first.
Malignant Thyroid Nodules:
> History of neck irradiation
> Fast-growing single, solid, and cold
> Dysphagia or hoarseness

Toxic Adenoma: Single palpable nodule with high radioactive uptake; the rest of the gland shows decreased uptake.

PARATHYROID GLAND DISORDERS

Hyperparathyroidism
Most cases are asymptomatic and are caused by a single adenoma.
Presentation: Bones, stones, moans, psychiatric overtones
Diagnostic Tests: Hypercalcemia, hypophosphatemia, and hypercalciuria
Treatment: Parathyroidectomy

ADRENAL GLAND DISORDERS

Addison's Disease (Primary Adrenal Insufficiency)
Caused by destruction of adrenal cortex; usually autoimmune in nature.
Presentation: Increased skin pigmentation, hyponatremia, and hyperkalemia
Diagnostic Tests: Elevated ACTH and decreased cortisol
Gold Standard: Short cosyntropin (ACTH) test
Treatment: Hydrocortisone and IV fluids

Secondary Adrenal Insufficiency
Most often due to previous use of corticosteroids (in as little as 4 weeks of steroid use).
Exogenous steroids suppress ACTH, allowing the adrenal gland to atrophy.
Presentation: Symptoms look like primary adrenal insufficiency without hyperpigmentation and hyponatremia.
Diagnostic Tests: Decreased ACTH and MSH, elevated cortisol, normal aldosterone
Treatment: Steroids and mineralocorticoids

Bones—bone pain and arthralgias

Stones—kidney stones

Moans—pancreatitis, or PUD

Psychiatric Overtones—depression, anxiety, irritability

Key: Unusual tan

Hyperadrenalism

Truncal obesity, moonlike facies, striae, poor wound healing, secondary diabetes, psychiatric disturbances, hypokalemia.

Cushing's Syndrome: Usually caused by prescribed steroids and is due to high cortisol levels

Cushing's Disease: Caused by pituitary overproduction of ACTH

Diagnostic Tests: First order 24-hour urine free cortisol and dexamethasone suppression test

ACTH-secreting pituitary adenomas—suppressed

Ectopic ACTH and adrenal cortisol tumors—not suppressed

If you suspect a lesion: CT of adrenal or MRI of brain to further localize

Treatment: Medical—mitotane; Surgical—resection or ablation depending on location

Conn's Syndrome (Primary Hyperaldosteronism)

Due to unilateral adrenal adenoma.

Presentation: Hypertension, muscle weakness, hypernatremia, hypokalemia, and *low renin*

Diagnostic Tests:

1. Measure plasma renin and aldosterone if consistent with primary hyperaldosteronism (hypernatremia, hypokalemia, elevated renin).
2. Confirm with aldosterone suppression test. Once confirmed:
3. CT of adrenal and look for mass.
4. If there is no mass on CT, do adrenal vein sampling.

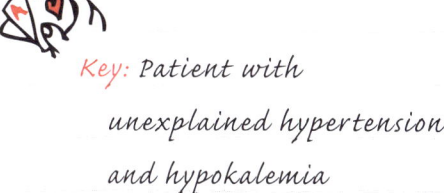

Key: Patient with unexplained hypertension and hypokalemia

Secondary Hyperaldosteronism

Labs may be variable.

Key Findings: High renin and presence of renal bruit

Pheochromocytoma

Chromaffin cell tumor that secretes epinephrine and norepinephrine.

Most common primary adrenal tumor in adults.

Presentation: Intermittent hypertension, tachycardia, feelings of impending doom

Diagnostic Tests: 24-hour urine for catecholamines; if positive order abdominal CT.

Treatment: First stabilize with alpha-blocker, followed by beta-blocker, then surgery.

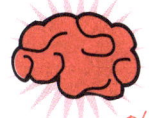

Pheochromocytoma

Follows Rule of 10s

- *10% familial*
- *10% in kids*
- *10% calcifications*
- *10% malignant*
- *10% bilateral*

Multiple Endocrine Neoplasia

MEN I (Wermer's Syndrome): Pituitary adenoma, pancreatic islet cell tumors, parathyroid adenoma

MEN II (Sipple's syndrome): Medullary thyroid CA, pheochromocytoma, parathyroid hyperplasia (increased PTH and Ca+)

MEN III (formerly MEN IIB): Medullary thyroid CA, pheochromocytoma, mucosal neuromas (tongue, eyelids, lip, GI), marfanoid habitus

Congenital Adrenal Hyperplasia

Congenital deficiency of cortisol.

Most commonly due to 21-hydroxylase deficiency.

Presentation: Ambiguous genitalia, precocious puberty, hypertension

Diagnostic Tests: Elevated cortisol precursors and androgens in urine and blood

Treatment: Cortisol administration reduces ACTH and adrenal androgens

DIABETES

Type I Diabetes Mellitus

Destruction of the beta cells of the pancreas leading to hyperglycemia secondary to insulin deficiency.

It is usually diagnosed in childhood and is autoimmune in origin.

Greatly decreased or absent insulin.

Associated with HLA-DR3 and -DR4.

Prone to DKA.

Presentation: Weight loss, polyuria, polydipsia, polyphagia

Need one of the following to make diagnosis:

1. Two separate occasions of fasting plasma glucose > 126 mg/dL
2. Two separate occasions of 2-hour postprandial glucose > 200 mg/dL after 75 g oral glucose tolerance test
3. Symptoms plus random plasma glucose > 200 mg/dL

Treatment: Insulin therapy; see Table 6-2.

HbA1c is used to monitor treatment and should be < 7.

TABLE 6-2 Insulin Therapy

Insulin Types	Onset	Peak	Duration
Fast-acting regular	30 min	4 hr	8 hr
Intermediate NPH lente	1–2 hr	4–12 hr	24 hr
Long-acting ultra lente	4 hr	10–30 hr	36 hr

DIABETIC KETOACIDOSIS

Seen in Type I DM only.

Anion gap metabolic acidosis

Cause: Infection or noncompliance

Treatment: Find underlying cause; insulin, fluids, NaCl, *potassium*, phosphate, bicarbonate

Type II Diabetes Mellitus

Reduced insulin secretion or increased insulin resistance.

Patients are commonly obese and over 40 years old.

No HLA type association.

Familial.

Susceptible to hyperlipidemia, hypertension.

Prone to hyperosmolar nonketotic coma.

(Presentation and diagnostic tests are the same as type I.)

Treatment: Weight reduction, metformin, glitazones, sulfonylureas, alpha-glucosidase inhibitors

HYPEROSMOLAR NONKETOTIC COMA

Seen in Type II DM only.

Mental status changes.

Treatment: Fluids

Hypoglycemia Symptoms: Lethargy, confusion, seizure, tachycardia, palpitations, tremor

See Table 6-3 for a list of diabetes complications.

POSTERIOR PITUITARY

Diabetes Insipidus

Patients have extreme polyuria and polydipsia.

CENTRAL VS NEPHROGENIC DIABETES INSIPIDUS

Central: Lack of ADH secretion from posterior pituitary; from trauma, neoplasm, or idiopathic

Nephrogenic: ADH insensitivity of the kidneys; usually induced by drugs (lithium, demeclocycline, methoxyflurane)

Diagnostic Tests: Administer ADH to differentiate between central and nephrogenic.

      Central: Responds to ADH

      Nephrogenic: Does not respond to ADH

Treatment:

      Central: Give ADH.

      Nephrogenic: Give thiazide diuretics.

Posterior Pituitary
- *Supraoptic releases— ADH*
- *Paraventricular releases—oxytocin*

SIADH

Water retention causing hyponatremia and other decreased electrolytes

Causes: Medications (morphine, chlorpropamide, oxytocin), small cell CA of lung, trauma, infection

Treatment: Water restriction

TABLE 6-3 Complications of Diabetes

Diabetic Retinopathy

Nonproliferative: Exudates, hemorrhage, microaneurysm
Treat with tight glucose control.
Proliferative: (~10% of patients) neovascularization
May cause vitreous hemorrhage and scar formation.
Can lead to acute blindness.
Treat with laser.

Diabetic Nephropathy

Kimmel-Steel-Wilson lesion
Papillary necrosis
Arteriosclerotic renal disease
Chronic interstitial nephritis
*Early marker—microalbuminuria and can progress to nephritic syndrome
Treat hypertension because it accelerates renal failure.
Decrease protein in diet.
Administer ACE inhibitor, which may help to slow progression.

Accelerated Atherosclerosis

Coronary artery disease (large and small)
Silent cardiac ischemia
Peripheral vascular disease in legs and feet
Small vessel disease may lead to foot infections, ulcers, gangrene, amputation.

Peripheral Neuropathy

If associated with pain, treat with gabapentin +/- TCAs.
Symmetric stocking and glove sensory loss
Numbness, tingling, burning
Treat with careful foot care

Autonomic Neuropathy

Gastroparesis
Postural hypotension
Urinary retention
Impotence in men

CHAPTER 7 GASTROINTESTINAL

This chapter is incredibly high yield. I cannot stress enough the importance of this chapter. You will see a large number of questions from this section. Why so many questions about GI? GI problems are found in all disciplines of medicine: surgery, pediatrics, gynecology, comorbid with other internal medicine pathologies, and even psychiatry (IBS). So, **learn it backward, forward, sideways; like it, love it, put it under your pillow and dream about it.**

ACHALASIA

Decreased or absent peristalsis of esophagus; increased pressure at LES
Dysphagia to solids *and* liquids
Diagnostic Test: Barium swallow shows bird beak narrowing
Confirmatory Test: Manometry
Treatment: Ca+ channel blockers, pneumatic dilatation, or surgical myomotomy

SCLERODERMA

Decreased peristalsis and incompetent LES sphincter
Diagnostic Test: Barium swallow
Confirmatory Test: Antitopoisomerase antibody
Dysphagia, reflux, plus CREST symptoms (Raynaud's symptoms are classically mentioned)
Complications: Peptic stricture; CREST—anticentromere antibodies

NUTCRACKER ESOPHAGUS

Classic motility disorder
Presentation: Chest pain due to strong erratic esophageal contractions
Diagnostic Test: Barium swallow shows "corkscrew" pattern
Confirmation Test: Manometric studies
Treatment: Ca+ channel blockers

Basic Rules for Esophageal Disorders

Dysphagia to solids = mechanical problem

Dysphagia to solids and liquids = motility problem

Progressive dysphagia to solids followed by liquids:

Tests: First-line—barium swallow

esophagoscopy, manometry, pH

If you suspect obstruction: Endoscopy and biopsy

Chest pain: Always rule out MI first, then consider

- *Esophageal motility disease: First-line test: contrast study (barium)*

- *Barium is standard unless GI perforation is suspected (use Gastrografin)*

Achalasia symptoms with history of travel to South America = Chaga's disease

MALLORY-WEISS TEAR

Superficial esophageal bleeding
Caused by repetitive vomiting (common in bulimics and skid
row alcoholics)
Diagnosis and Treatment: Endoscopy

BOERHAAVE'S TEAR

Full thickness esophageal tear; can be complication of
above or endoscopy
Treatment: Surgical emergency

ZENKER DIVERTICULUM

Out-pouching of esophagus where food gets trapped
Presentation: Halitosis that could curl your hair!
Conformational Test: Barium esophagogram

ESOPHAGEAL CANCER

*Barrett's or GERD =
Adenocarcinoma
Smoking and Alcohol =
Squamous Cell Carcinoma*

Upper esophagus—squamous cell carcinoma is most
common.
Lower esophagus—adenocarcinoma associated with
Barrett's esophagus (changes from squamous to
columnar caused by GERD).

HIATAL HERNIAS

Sliding type: Common and benign; GE junction slides above
diaphragm
Paraesophageal: Portion of fundus herniates above
diaphragm; GE junction remains below

GASTROESOPHAGEAL REFLUX DISEASE (GERD)

Decreased lower esophageal sphincter pressure or increased
frequency in LES relaxation
Decreased esophageal peristalsis
Caustic material reflux
Retarded gastric emptying
Presentation: Chest pain (rule out MI), dysphagia, cough,
hoarseness, heartburn
Key: Eat, lay supine = heartburn or new onset nocturnal
asthma

Tests:
1. Esophagoscopy
2. 24-hour pH

Increased incidence in patients with sliding type hiatal hernia

Complications: Stricture and Barrett's esophagus—transformation from squamous to columnar epithelium (Barrett's esophagus carries increased risk of esophageal adenocarcinoma.)

Treatment: Antacids, PPIs, H2 blockers, and advise to avoid exacerbating factors; surgery for cases that do not respond to therapy

PEPTIC ULCER DISEASE (PUD)

Epigastric tenderness and pain

Presentation: Epigastric pain and tenderness; awaken with epigastric pain with or without nausea and vomiting; possible blood in stool (upper or lower in origin) or obstruction

Diagnostic Tests:
1. Barium swallow
2. Breath test and blood serology (diagnostic)
3. Endoscopy with biopsy

Treatment: H2 blocker, PPIs, antacids, and *H. pylori* detection and eradication plus amoxicillin, clarithromycin

Refractory to treatment—surgery

Complications: Perforation (chemical peritonitis) = Boardlike abdomen with free air on x-ray

Two Types of Peptic Ulcer Disease: Gastric and Duodenal

Gastric: Commonly caused by NSAIDs; associated with blood type A

Duodenal: Vast majority of cases of PUD; associated with *H. pylori* infection; associated with blood type O

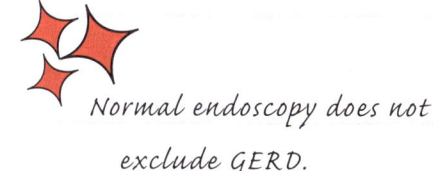

Normal endoscopy does not exclude GERD.

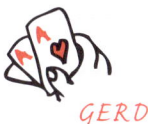

GERD

Exacerbating Factors: Anticholinergic meds, alcohol, smoking, spicy food, coffee, chocolate

Always biopsy gastric ulcers to rule out gastric cancer!

Elevated serum gastrin levels should alert you to consider Zollinger-Ellison syndrome

Aprostol is contraindicated in pregnant patients.

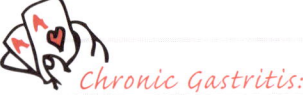

Chronic Gastritis:

Type A (rare)—Autoimmune

    Antiparietal cell antibodies

Type B (most common)—

    Helicobacter Infection

    Antrum of stomach

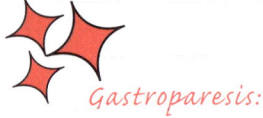

Gastroparesis:

Commonly associated with DM

Stomach Cancer:

Virchow's node—Left

    supraclavicular node

Krukenberg tumor—ovarian

    METS from stomach CA

Conjugated bilirubin elevated

    more than unconjugated

    bilirubin

Clay stool and dark urine

Jaundice and pruritis

Suspect problem in common

    bile duct—ERCP

Confirm problems in common

    bile duct—Cholangiogram

Acute Cholecystitis:

Five Fs: Female, Fat, 40,

    Fertile, Flatulent

GASTRITIS

Nausea and vomiting and/or hematemesis
Stomach lining inflammation
Diagnostic Test: Endoscopy
Acute Gastritis: Severe injury-induced stress, NSAIDs
Chronic Gastritis: Type A and Type B

GASTROPARESIS

Bloating, distension, pain, early satiety, weight loss
Diagnostic Test: Gastric emptying scan
Treatment: Cisapride (prolongs QT interval), erythromycin
Most common complication is hemorrhage.

STOMACH CANCER

Risk Factors: Japanese, smoking, high nitrites, *H. pylori*
    infection, chronic gastritis
Diagnostic Test: Endoscopy and biopsy

CARCINOID TUMOR

Symptoms usually don't begin until CA metastasizes.
Carcinoid Syndrome: Abdominal cramps, diarrhea, skin
    flushing
Labs: 5-HIAA increased in urine

BILE DUCT OBSTRUCTION

Diseases of the Gallbladder
Risk Factors: Hemolysis (pigmented stones), birth control
    pills, Native American origin

Cholelithiasis
Transient blockage of cystic duct
Presentation: RUQ pain after a fatty meal that may radiate to
    scapula; with or without nausea, vomiting, and jaundice
Diagnostic Test: U/S or upper GI series to rule out hiatal
    hernia or ulcer
Treatment: Cholecystectomy

Acute Cholecystitis
Prolonged cystic duct blockage that leads to inflammation
    of the gallbladder

Presentation: Fever, RUQ pain, Murphy sign
Diagnostic Test: U/S or positive HIDA if gallbladder is not
visualized
Treatment: Antibiotics, ERCP, cholecystectomy; if diabetic,
cool down infection and wait 4–6 hours before surgery

Choledocholithiasis
Blockage of common bile duct
Increased alkaline phosphatase and total bilirubin
Treatment: ERCP and stone removal

ACUTE CHOLANGITIS

Biliary tree infection
Increased alkaline phosphatase and bilirubin
Cause: Choledocholithiasis or primary sclerosing cholangitis
(young person with IBD)
Diagnostic and Therapuetic: ERCP

PRIMARY BILIARY CIRRHOSIS

Antimitochondrial antibodies
Presentation: Jaundiced, itchy woman; may have fat-soluble
vitamin deficiency
Diagnostic Tests: Increased alk phos or GGT with or without
mild elevation of AST ALT
Treatment: Cholestyramine helps symptoms but does not
cure; liver transplant is curative.

PRIMARY SCLEROSING CHOLANGITIS

Associated with inflammatory bowel disease plus jaundice
and pruritis
Similar lab values as primary biliary cirrhosis
Diagnostic Tests: ERCP—bile duct stricture/bleeding
15% develop cholangiosarcoma

MUCOCELE

Thickened gallbladder wall
See Figure 7-1 to see disorders associated with anatomical
positions.

*Causes of Increased Alkaline
Phosphatase:*
*Obstructive biliary tract
disease*
METS to bone
Paget's disease (bone)

*90% of gallstones found in
cystic duct; 10% in common
bile duct*

*Bile duct appears normal on
U/S.*

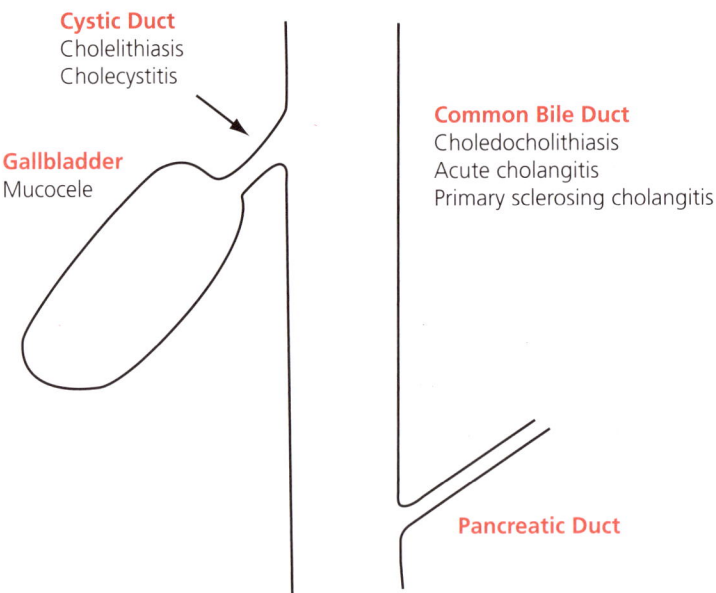

FIGURE 7-1 Gastrointestinal Anatomy

Cystic Duct
Cholelithiasis
Cholecystitis

Gallbladder
Mucocele

Common Bile Duct
Choledocholithiasis
Acute cholangitis
Primary sclerosing cholangitis

Pancreatic Duct

All hepatitis labs show increased ALT/AST, bilirubin, and alk phos. Diagnosis for all hepatitis is made by serology.

LIVER DISEASE

Hepatitis A

30-day incubation period
Fecal oral transmission
Diagnostic Tests: HAV IgM
Anti-HAV IgM means previous exposure and lifelong
  immunity
Never chronic
Exposure: Chronic liver disease or travel to endemic areas
Immunize with human Ig
Treatment: Supportive

Hepatitis B

3-month incubation period
Transmissible through DNA, blood
Carries increased risk for hepatocellular carcinoma
Diagnostic Tests:
- HBs Ag (acute or chronic infection)
- HBc Ab—IgM window phase
- HBe Ag—measure of infectivity

Exposure: Vaccine plus HBIg
Treatment:
  Acute: Supportive
  Chronic: Alpha IFN plus lamuvidine

After liver transplant to prevent recurrent HBV
infection: HBIg + lamuvidine

Hepatitis C

The hepatitis you get after a transfusion or sharing needles.
Associated with lichen planus.
Anti-HCV is not a useful marker in the acute phase.
Asymptomatic patients will show increased transaminases.
90% of cases evolve to chronic.
Treatment:
Acute: IFN-alpha and ribavirin
Chronic: IFN-beta and ribavirin

Hepatitis D

Only exists as coinfection with hep B
Superinfection in chronic carrier
Key: Mostly seen in IVDU and hemophiliacs

Hepatitis E

Epidemic in some parts of Asia
Fecal oral transmission
Hep D Ag-IgM Ab—recent resolution to infection
Hep D antigen alone—chronicity
Key: Fulminant disease in pregnancy

Autoimmune Hepatitis

Anti–smooth muscle or antinuclear antibodies
Presentation: Young woman with or without other
autoimmune disease
Treatment: Azathioprine, steroids

Liver biopsy to distinguish between chronic active hepatitis and chronic persistent hepatitis

Manifestations of Chronic Liver Disease and Liver Failure

- Jaundice
- Spider nevi
- Gynecomastia
- Hypoglycemia
- Elevated conjugated and unconjugated bilirubin
- Portal hypertension—hemorrhoids, varices (melena and hematemesis)
- Bleeding problems: Give fresh frozen plasma because damaged livers cannot use vitamin K
- Ascites: Treat underlying liver disease, diuretics, decreased salt intake

- Spontaneous bacterial peritonitis: Complication of ascites; infected perotineal fluid that can progress to sepsis

Diagnostic Tests: Paracentesis to obtain fluid sample and WBC, Gram stain, protein, glucose

Treatment: IV antibiotics

- Hyperammonemia that leads to hepatic encephalopathy

Treat by decreasing all sources of ammonia: Normal flora make ammonia (give neomycin), decrease protein intake, lactulose (prevents ammonia absorption).

Portal Hypertension
Portal pressure > 12 mmHg

Presentation: Jaundice, ascites, mental status changes, esophageal varices; may present as spontaneous bacterial peritonitis

B-blocker to prevent bleeds and rebleeds

Dubin-Johnson Syndrome
AR elevated conjugated bilirubin

Presentation: Commonly asymptomatic

Jaundice exacerbated by pregnancy, BCPs, or infection

Hemachromatosis
AR inheritance (onset: around 45 years old)

Hyperabsorption of iron

Cause can be secondary to chronic transfusion therapy (seen in beta thalassemics) or alcoholism

Presentation: Abdo pain, DM, hypogonadism, cirrhosis, bronze skin, CHF, anemia

Diagnostic Tests: Serum iron studies will exhibit increased iron, saturation, ferritin, and greatly increased transferrin.

Associated with pseudogout.

Confirmatory Tests: Fasting transferrin, liver biopsy

Treatment: Deferoxamine and serial phlebotomy

Wilson's Disease
AR chromosome 13 deficient copper transporters

Affects basal ganglia

Presentation: Mental status changes, choreiform movements, asterixis, Kayser-Fleischer rings

Diagnostic Tests: Decreased ceruloplasmin and increased copper deposition in liver and brain

Treatment: Ceruloplasmin and copper dietary restriction

Hepatocellular Carcinoma (Hepatoma)
Caused by cirrhosis and chronic hepatitis
Presentation: RUQ pain, jaundice, ascites, coagulopathy
Diagnostic Tests: Mass on CT/US plus increased LFTs and AFP
Spreads hematogenously
Confirmatory Test: Liver biopsy
Treatment: Transplant
Check AFP levels to monitor recurrence.

See Table 7-1 for review and additional information on liver disease.

TABLE 7-1 Facts About Liver Disease

Causes
Cholestasis—commonly caused by pregnancy or medications
Reye's Syndrome—suspect in a child with viral-induced fever who has taken aspirin
Hepatic adenoma—caused by BCPs
Cholangiosarcoma—caused by UC or clonorchis liver fluke
Angiosarcoma—caused by vinyl exposure

Histology
Councilman's bodies in liver—yellow fever
Mallory bodies in liver—alcoholic

Associations
Budd-Chiari syndrome—associated with PRV
Third-trimester-pregnant patient that develops fatty liver—treatment is delivery
Alpha-1 antitrypsin deficiency—young person with emphysema and cirrhosis
Patient with asymptomatic elevation of aminotransferase—Always rule out alcohol, drug use, and risk factors for hepatitis.
Hepatocellular carcinoma (hepatoma)—increased AFP

Hepatitis
Liver biopsy—distinguish chronic active vs chronic persistent hepatitis
Hep B and Hep C can turn into chronic hepatitis.
Hep B and Hep C are associated with increased incidence of hepatic cancer.
Alcoholic hepatitis—AST > ALT, 2:1
Autoimmune hepatitis—anti–smooth muscle or antinuclear Abs

Angiodysplasia is associated with aortic stenosis.

Meckel's Rule of 2s

2 years old

2:1, male:female predominance

2 types of mucosa involved

2 feet from ileocecal valve

UPPER GI BLEED VS LOWER GI BLEED

Distinction point is ligament of Treitz.

Presentation:
> Upper—tarry dark stool (melena)
> Lower—bright red blood in stool

Diagnostic Tests: NG tube followed by endoscopy (upper or lower)
> Very slow bleed detection—labeled erythrocyte scintigraphy
> Slow bleed detection—radionuclide scan
> Fast bleed detection—angiography

Angiodysplasia

Elderly patient with a lower GI bleed

Presentation: Painless lower GI bleeding in the elderly

Diagnostic Tests: Endoscopy; if unsure after endoscopy, perform a labeled erythrocyte scintigraphy

Meckel's Diverticulum

Child with lower GI bleed

Presentation: Painless rectal bleeding

Diagnostic Test: Technetium scan

Mesenteric Ischemia

Atherosclerosis of superior mesenteric artery

Presentation: History of pain after eating, which leads to significant weight loss
> Patient will commonly have extensive atherosclerotic disease (current or in history).

Key: Pain out of proportion to physical exam findings

Acidosis, hyperkalemia, leukocytosis

Diagnostic Test: CT scan reveals thickening of bowel wall

Confirmatory Test: Angiogram

Treatment: Surgery

Ischemic Colitis

Inferior mesenteric artery

Usually due to low flow—splenic flexure and rectosigmoid
vasculature "watershed area"

May follow AAA or IMA damage

Presentation: Painless bleeding; bloody diarrhea and pain

Left-sided abdominal findings

Abnormal abdo x-ray

Diagnostic Test: Angiogram (early)

Diverticulosis

Most common cause of lower GI bleed in elderly

Caused by herniation of mucosa in intestinal wall (usually in
sigmoid colon)

Risk Factors: Low-fiber, high-fat diet

Presentation: Painless rectal bleeding, LLQ pain, diarrhea or
constipation

Treatment:

Mild bleeding—increase fiber intake

Moderate bleeding—watch; angiography with
embolization if needed

Diverticulitis

Acute LLQ pain, nausea and vomiting, increased WBC count

Diagnostic Test: CT scan

Treatment: NPO and antibiotics

Sigmoidoscopy carries risk for perforation in patients with diverticulitis.

Colon Cancer

See Table 7-2.

Always suspect in: Middle-aged patient with occult blood
in stool

Presentation: Relatively asymptomatic, or over 40 years
old with rectal bleeding and/or anemia with change in
bowel habits or stool caliber

Diagnostic Tests: CBC, stool for guaiac; sigmoidoscopy
detects left-sided lesion; colonoscopy detects right-sided
lesion

Investigation should include looking for METS.

Treatment: Surgery or surgery plus chemotherapy (if nodes
test positive)

Left-sided lesion—Apple core lesion and change in bowel habits

Right-sided lesion—Anemia and change in stool caliber

Always remove and examine all polyps.

Marker for colon cancer: CEA
(not used for screening)

1. *Measure preoperatively*
2. *Remove cancer*
3. *Measure postoperatively*

CEA should decrease

Any increase in CEA
postoperatively =
reoccurrence

Malignant Potential of Polyps
(from most to least):
Villous > Tubular > Sessile
> Pedunculated

Inflammatory Bowel Disease
(See Table 7-3)

Ulcerative Colitis vs Crohn's
Disease

Initial presentation seen in
young people

Diagnostic Tests: Barium
Proctosigmoidoscopy + Biopsy

TABLE 7-2 Facts About Colon Cancer

Colon Cancer Facts
Most common first sign of colon cancer is rectal bleeding.
ANYONE over 40 years old with rectal bleeding: ALWAYS suspect colon cancer.
Colon cancer—#1 cause of large bowel obstruction in adults.
#2 cause of cancer deaths.
Colon Cancer Risk Factors
Age
History of ulcerative colitis > Crohn's disease
Family history
High-fat, low-fiber diet
Colon Cancer Screening
"Birthday gifts that start at 50 years old"
Annual DRE with stool guaiac test
Every 3–5 years sigmoidoscopy
Every 10 years colonoscopy
Colonoscopy in patients more than 40 years old with family history

TABLE 7-3 Inflammatory Bowel Disease

Ulcerative Colitis	Crohn's Disease
Key: More common in Jewish people	**Key:** Nephrolithiasis, fistulas
Involves colon 　Rectum	Involves colon—bloody diarrhea 　Ileum—mimics appendicitis
Bloody diarrhea, toxic megacolon	Watery diarrhea, perianal fistulas, abscesses
Other symptoms: Sclerosis cholangitis, sacroileitis, erythema nodosum, peripheral arthritis	Other symptoms: Same as UC plus fistulas to urinary tract, nephrolithiasis
Lesions: Continuous symmetric	Lesions: Skip
Mucosal inflammation	Transmural inflammation
Pseudopolyps	Noncaseating granulomas
Barium: Short lead pipe colon	Barium: Transverse fissures
Greatly increased cancer risk	Slightly increased cancer risk
Treatment: Sulfasalazine, topical mesalamine, steroids	Treatment: Sulfasalazine, steroids
Surgery is curative.	Surgery is therapeutic, NOT curative.

No onset of ulcerative colitis and Crohn's disease in old age; therefore, if you see an elderly patient with inflammatory bowel symptoms, consider pseudomembranous or ischemic colitis.

IRRITABLE BOWEL SYNDROME

Change in bowel habits related to stress levels
Commonly presents as pattern of alternating periods of diarrhea and constipation
Most commonly seen with coexisting anxiety or depression
Diagnostic Test: Diagnosis of exclusion
Treatment: Antidiarrheal meds

MALABSORPTION

Associated with fat-soluble vitamin deficiency (A, D, E, K)
Presentation: Fat-soluble vitamin deficiency, greasy stool, weight loss, coagulation problems, and anemia
Labs will show: Low calcium, iron, folate, and B_{12}

D-xylose test is a good test to prove that the pancreas is normal but the small bowel is abnormal.

Diagnosis: Biopsy shows villous atrophy, positive antiendomysial antibodies, and abnormal D-xylose test.

Dermatitis herpetiformis = rash on thighs

Diagnostic Tests for All Malabsorption Syndromes

1. 48- to 72-hour stool fecal fat collection: positive sudan black stain
2. D-xylose test—measures absorption ability of the small intestine
3. Small bowel biopsy

Celiac Disease and Other Malabsorption Syndromes

CELIAC DISEASE
Chronic sensitivity to gluten (wheat, barley, rye)
Effects proximal small bowel
Presentation: Symptoms of malabsorption plus iron deficiency
Treatment: Exclude gluten from diet
Dermatitis herpetiformis—associated with celiac sprue
Rash treatment: Dapsone

WHIPPLE'S DISEASE
Caused by *Tropheryma whippelii*, which is a Gram positive bacillus
Presentation: Looks like celiac disease plus CNS symptoms and arthralgias
Diagnostic Test: Small bowel biopsy histology shows foamy macrophages with PAS stain
Treatment: Sulfa drug or tetracycline for a duration of 6 months–1 year

TROPICAL SPRUE
Looks like celiac disease with history of travel to the tropics: South America, Caribbean, or India
Primarily affects the ileum
Causes B_{12} deficiency
Diagnostic Test: Biopsy
Treatment: Sulfa drug or tetracycline for 4–6 months plus folate

DIARRHEA

(See also Chapter 10, "Infectious Disease," and Chapter 14, "Pediatrics.")

Shigella
Dysentery with blood and mucous

Consider shigella in the following scenarios:
Kid with new seizure or bloody diarrhea in an institutionalized patient

Clostridium Difficile (Non-IBD Colitis)
Presentation: Watery diarrhea in hospitalized patient after taking antibiotics—clindamycin, cephalosporins, ampicillin
Diagnostic Test: C-diff toxin assay
Pseudomembranes seen with flexible sigmoidoscopy.

Campylobacter
Resembles ulcerative colitis

Consider campylobacter if question includes: UC symptoms after a suspect meal with or without reactive arthritis.

Giardia Lamblia
Steatorrhea plus protozoal cysts in stool
Above symptoms plus history of camping and drinking spring water
Diagnostic Test: Duodenal aspirate
Treatment: Metronidazole

Entamoeba Histolytica
Can have up to a 3-month incubation period
Presentation: Traveler's diarrhea
Diagnostic Tests: Culture, biopsy, serology
Treatment: Metronidazole

Traveler's Diarrhea
ETEC *E. coli*
Severe watery diarrhea; without blood or fever
Treatment: Antibiotics, loperamide

Yersinia Enterocolitica
Diarrhea plus acute onset RLQ pain
Diagnostic Tests: Stool culture, serology

See Table 7-4 for the differences between small bowel obstruction and large bowel obstruction.

"Appendicitis-like" pain

When you see E. coli and/or shigella diarrhea, always consider "HUTS" Hemolytic uremic syndrome.

Any older patient with

abdominal symptoms:

Always screen for colon CA!

TABLE 7-4 Small Bowel Obstruction vs Large Bowel Obstruction

Small Bowel Obstruction: Hyperactive bowel sounds, abdominal distension, bilious vomiting

Diagnostic Test: Abdominal x-ray shows stepladder appearance or multi-air fluid levels

In adults = Adhesions (with history of prior surgery)

In children = Intussusception or incarcerated hernia

Treatment: NPO, NG tube, IV fluids, and observation

If no improvement *within 24 hours* or fever and leukocytes develop, then **surgery**

Large Bowel Obstruction: Abdominal pain and distension, constipation, feculent vomiting

In adults = Diverticulitis, volvulus (can be decompressed with endoscope), colon cancer

In children = Hirschsprung's disease

Other causes:

- Sigmoid volvulus: Treat with barium enema.
- Paralytic ileus: Loss of intestinal peristalsis without structural obstruction; treat with bethenachol.

PANCREAS

Acute Pancreatitis

Caused By: Alcohol, gallstones, trauma, hypertrigly-ceridemia, hyperkalemia, steroids, mumps, scorpion sting, or drugs

Presentation: Abdominal pain that "bores through" to back, plus nausea and vomiting

Diagnostic Tests: Increased amylase and lipase

Confirmation Tests: U/S or CT scan

Treatment: Meperimide (because it doesn't tighten sphincter of Odie) NPO, fluids, fat-soluble vitamins and enzyme replacement

Complications: Pancreatic pseudocyst (suspect if you see increased serum and urine amylase)

Increased phospholipase—can cause ARDS

See Table 7-5 for Ranson's criteria for acute pancreatitis.

Cullen's sign—Black and blue

umbilicus

Grey-Turner's sign—Black and

blue flanks

TABLE 7-5 Ranson's Criteria for Acute Pancreatitis

On Admission	Age > 50 years old
	Glucose > 200 mg/dL
	LDH > 350 IU/dL
	AST > 250 IU/dL
	WBC > 16,000/mL
2 Days After Onset	PaO_2 < 60 mmHG
	Calcium < 8.0 mg/dL
	Sequestered fluid > 6 L
	HCT drops by > 10%
	Base excess > 4 mEq/L
	BUN increase > 5 mg/dL

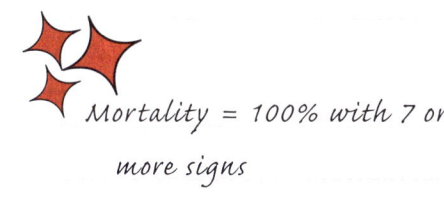

Mortality = 100% with 7 or more signs

Chronic Pancreatitis
Alcoholic with recurrent episodes of pancreatitis
Diagnosis: Calcification of pancreas on x-ray
Treatment: Stop drinking, pain management

Vipoma
Pancreatic cholera
Diagnostic Test: CT scan

Glucagonoma
Most common in females and most commonly malignant
Affects alpha cells
Presentation: DM-like symptoms with skin lesions on
 extremities; hyperglycemia with highly elevated
 glucagon and necrotizing erythematous skin lesions

Zollinger-Ellison Syndrome
Multiple peptic ulcers with elevated acid secretion and
 gastrinoma
Diagnostic Test: Serum gastrin levels

Insulinoma
Hypoglycemia plus CNS symptoms
Affects beta cells
Diagnostic Test: Check C-peptide to rule out DM
Key: Elevated C-peptide
Treatment: Glucose to relieve symptoms; resection is
 curative

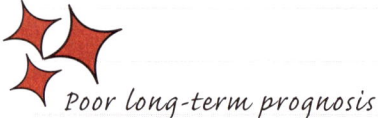

Poor long-term prognosis

Pancreatic Cancer

Starts from ductal epithelium in head of pancreas

Presentation: Elderly patient with obstructive jaundice, pain, and weight loss

- Most important risk factor—smoking
- Courvoisier's sign—palpable, nontender gallbladder
- Trousseau's sign—migratory thrombophlebitis

Diagnostic Tests: CT scan, ERCP, FNA

Treatment: Primarily palliative; or Whipple procedure

CHAPTER 8 GYNECOLOGY

BREAST CANCER

Breast cancer is the most common cancer to afflict women and the second most common cause of cancer death.

Presentation of Breast CA: Palpable lump or detected by mammogram

Most common location is upper outer quadrant.

Hard, painless, immobile lump

Other possible features: Skin changes, adenopathy in axilla, nipple discharge

For breast cancer diagnostic tests, see Figure 8-1.

FIGURE 8-1 Diagnostic Tests

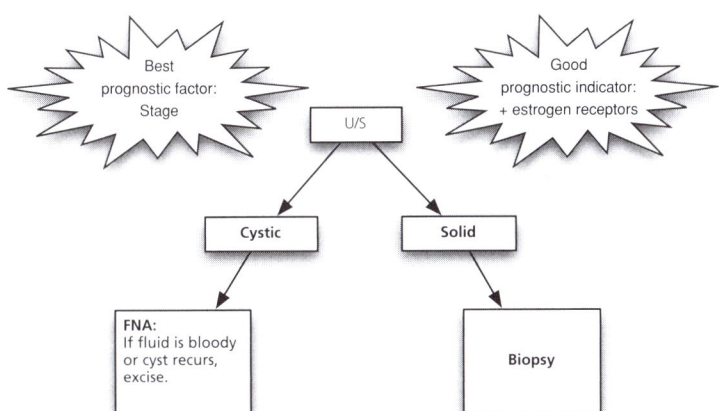

Tamoxifen

Treats tumors with positive estrogen status, give to all patients with axillary METS; decreases mortality by preventing recurrences and development in opposite breast.

Side Effects: Vaginal dryness and hot flashes

BENIGN BREAST DISEASE

Fibrocystic Change

Premenopausal women with nodular, bilateral, cyclic breast tenderness

Diagnostic Tests: FNA and cytology

Breast Cancer Screening

35–40 years old—
Baseline mammogram

40–50 years old—
Mammogram every 2 years

50 years old and older—
Annual mammogram

Mammogram is not diagnostic in lactating women or women under 20 years old.

Risk Factors for Breast Cancer

Increased estrogen exposure = Increased breast CA

Early menarche, late menopause, nulliparity, or late first-time pregnancy

Female gender, family or personal history of breast CA, old age

Remember:

Lobular Carcinoma: Increased risk of being bilateral

Paget's Disease: Nipple erosion

Intraductal Papilloma: Bloody nipple discharge

Most common breast mass in women under 30 years old

Typical Commonly Tested Patterns of Breast Disease

Found only during lactation (breast feeding): Breast Abscess

20-year-old with rubbery movable mass: Fibroadenoma

Benign, fast-growing fibroadenoma: Phyllodes Tumor

Malignant, fast growing: Cystosarcoma Phyllodes

30-year-old with nodular lumps that change with cycle: Fibrocystic Change

Endometrial cancer must be ruled out in any case of abnormal vaginal bleeding in postmenopausal women.

Fibroadenoma

Movable, round, rubbery mass

Diagnostic Test and Treatment: Surgical excision

ABNORMAL VAGINAL BLEEDING

Premenarche Vaginal Bleeding

Most common cause is foreign body or trauma.

VAGINAL OR CERVICAL CANCER (SARCOMA BOTRYOIDES)

Presents as "bunch of grapes" hanging out of cervix or vagina

PRECOCIOUS PUBERTY

Presents as vaginal bleeding, pubic hair, and breast development before onset of puberty. Average onset of puberty is around 9 years old with breast development. The most common cause of precocious puberty is idiopathic, but tumor, adrenal lesions, and all other diagnoses must be ruled out before deeming the cause idiopathic.

Treatment: Leuprolide, a GNRH analogue, down regulates the pituitary gland; treatment is an imperative. Without treatment premature epiphyseal closure can occur.

MCCUNE-ALBRIGHT SYNDROME

Precocious puberty, pigmentation, polyostotic fibrous dysplasia

Postmenarche Vaginal Bleeding

Vaginal atrophy is the most common cause.

Treatment: HRT

Diagnostic Test: D&C

Abnormal Bleeding During Reproductive Age

Pregnancy is the most common cause of abnormal bleeding in reproductive-age women. HCG is *always* the first test to order in this scenario.

Diagnostic Test: B-HCG

See Figure 8-2 for additional information on abnormal vaginal bleeding.

FIGURE 8-2 Abnormal Vaginal Bleeding

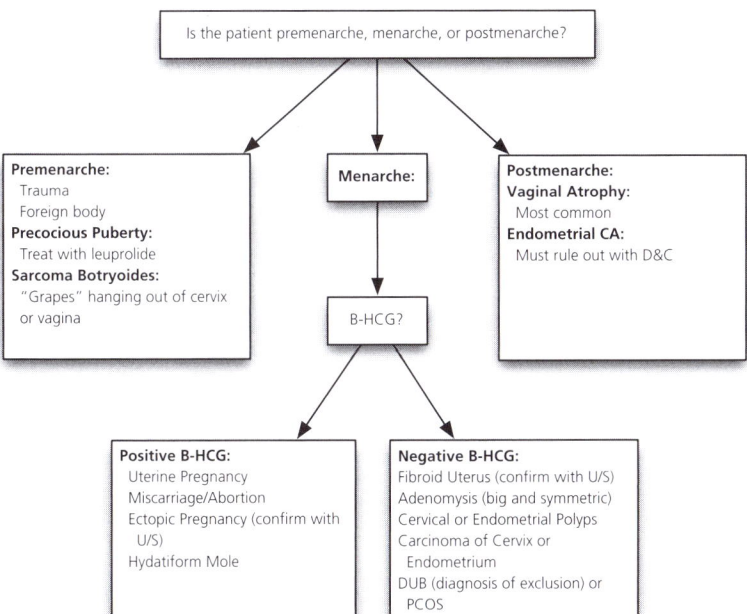

Referred shoulder pain is associated with ectopic pregnancy.

Risk Factors for Ectopic Pregnancy

Previous tubal or pelvic surgery

DES exposure in utero

IUD use

Most Common: Previous PID infection

If ectopic:

Is less than 3.5 cm

No fetal heart tones heard

B-HCG less than 1500 mIU/mL

Treatment: Methotrexate (folate is contraindicated)

If ectopic pregnancy *does not* meet criteria, surgical intervention is needed: salpingostomy or salpingectomy and *give RhoGAM to all Rh− women.*

Hydatiform mole—benign

Choriocarcinoma—malignant

Two in ten hydatiform moles develop choriocarcinoma.

POSITIVE B-HCG

Ectopic Pregnancy

Most common location for implantation is ampulla of oviduct.

1% incidence rate.

Presentation: Amenorrhea, pelvic or abdominal pain, plus light vaginal bleeding

Ruptured Ectopic Presentation: Sudden onset, sharp abdominal pain with rebound tenderness or may present as shock

Diagnostic Tests: B-HCG then U/S

Transabdominal U/S if B-HCG is more than 5000 mIU/mL

Transvaginal U/S if B-HCG is less than 1500–2000 mIU/mL

Definitive Diagnosis: U/S *visualization* or laparoscopy

Gestational Trophoblastic Disease

Placenta develops tumor

Complete Mole: 46 XX (sperm plus empty ovum), paternally derived and contains no fetal parts

Incomplete Mole: 69 XXY (two sperm plus normal ovum), may contain some fetal parts

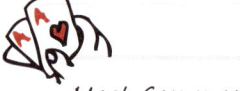

Most Common Mole

   Presentation:

HCG very high

Uterus very large

Hypertension early in

   pregnancy

Possible hyperthyroidism or

   adnexal mass

If B-HCG continues to rise, the

mole is choriocarcinoma.

Order CT to look for

METS and treat with

chemotherapy.

Diagnostic Test: U/S shows "snowstorm pattern"

Treatment: First, suction curettage; next, put patient on oral contraceptive pills and follow B-HCG levels until 0.

Abortion

See Table 8-1 for types of abortion and their treatment.

TABLE 8-1 Types of Abortion and Their Treatment

	Symptoms	Signs	U/S	Treatment
Threatened Abortion	Minimal bleeding and cramping	Cervical os closed (most common cause is abnormal karyotype)	Normal	Conservative
Missed Abortion	No bleeding and cramping	Cervical os closed	No viable pregnancy	D&C; if mother is Rh− give RhoGAM
	Bleeding and cramping	Cervical os dilated but no tissue has passed		Emergency D&C; if mother is Rh− give RhoGAM
Incomplete Abortion	Bleeding and cramping	Cervical os dilated, some tissue has passed and some remains		Emergency D&C; if mother is Rh− give RhoGAM
Complete Abortion	Bleeding and cramping (but now minimal)	Cervical os dilated, has passed tissue and nothing remains	Normal uterine stripe	Observation

NEGATIVE B-HCG

Adenomyosis

Large symmetric uterus

Diagnostic Test: U/S and size uterus like a pregnant uterus

Fibroid Uterus (Uterine Leiomyoma)
More common in African American females over 35 years old
Presentation: Abnormal bleeding, commonly painful, anemia, infertility
Estrogen Dependent: *Regresses after menopause, larger with pregnancy*
Diagnostic Test: U/S and size like pregnant uterus
Treatment: GNRH analogues can shrink fibroids, but their postmenopausal side effects are not well tolerated.

Causes of Abnormal Bleeding

PERMANENT: PCOS
Bilateral polycystic ovaries with symptoms caused by increased androgens
Presentation: Anovulatory cycles = infertility; increased LH and androgens = obesity and hirsutism
> Associated symptoms: insulin resistance and diabetes.
> Increased, unopposed estrogen = increased risk of endometrial cancer.
> Hirsutism is caused by increased levels of testosterone.

Diagnostic Tests: U/S shows bilateral polycystic ovaries, LH/FSH > 2:1, increased serum DHEA
Treatment: Oral contraceptive pills, infertility responds to clomiphene

TEMPORARY: DUB
Diagnosis of exclusion; all other possibilities must be ruled out
Treatment: Progesterone day 14–25, or oral contraceptive pills

Pelvic exam = Firm, "Lumpy Bumpy Uterus"

If grows after menopause, not a fibroid

Treatment if patient still wants children? Myomectomy
Does not still want children? Hysterectomy

Anovulation is usually caused by stress.

AMENORRHEA

For explanations and definitions of amenorrhea, see Figure 8-3.

FIGURE 8-3 Amenorrhea

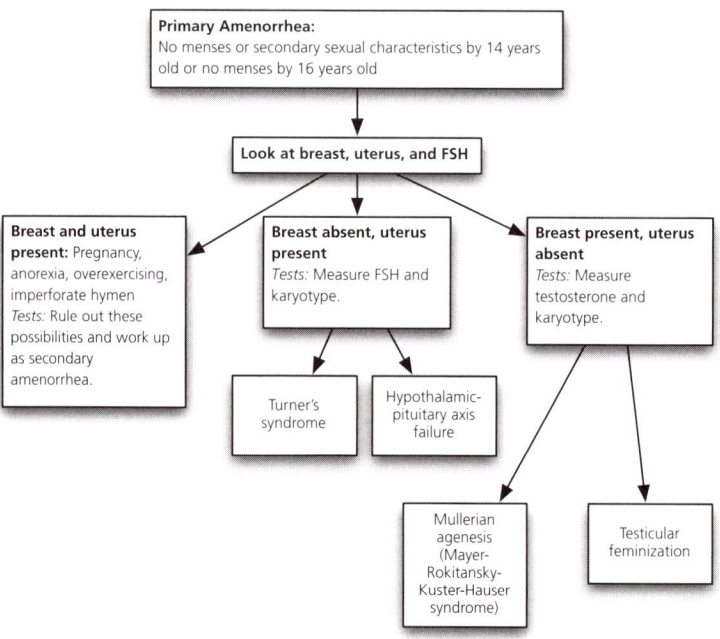

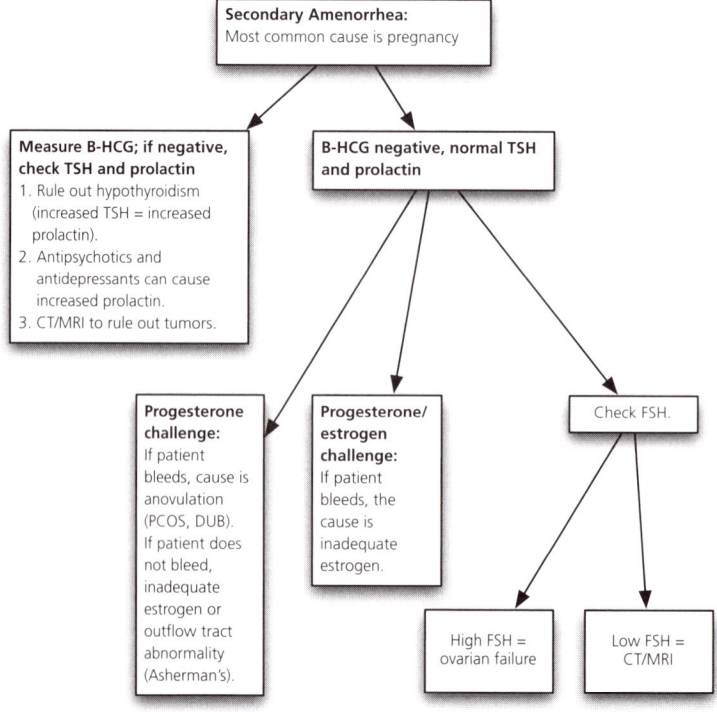

MENOPAUSE

Average age: around 51 years old; smoking = earlier menopausal age

Presentation: Irregular menstrual cycle, mood changes, hot flashes, vaginal atrophy/dryness, dysuria

Diagnostic Test: Increased FSH and absent menses for 1 year

Treatment: HRT, always use combined progesterone/ estrogen

Contraindications for HRT: History of breast or endometrial cancer, thrombosis, liver disease, undiagnosed vaginal bleeding

If patient refuses HRT: To prevent osteoporosis, give Ca+, vit D, biphosphonates, estrogen cream for vaginal atrophy

Early Menopause: Menopause before 40 years old

DYSMENORRHEA

Severe pain with menstruation

Primary Dysmenorrhea
Common before 20 years old
Possible Cause: Elevated PGs and leukotrienes
Treatment: NSAIDs and BCPs

Secondary Dysmenorrhea
Pain with menstruation is second to pathology of pelvis.

ENDOMETRIOSIS
Ectopic endometrial glands
Most common secondary cause of dysmenorrhea
Presentation: Pain with sex (dyspareunia), pain with defecation (dyschezia), premenstrual pain, *infertility*
Pelvic Exam: Reveals nodules on uterosacral ligament, retroverted uterus
Diagnostic Test: Laparoscopy of ectopic tissue— appears like chocolate cysts and powder burns
Treatment: Oral contraceptive pills, danazol (not well tolerated), or surgery (laparoscopic ablation or hysterectomy)

Estrogen alone is acceptable only if patient had total hysterectomy.

Estrogen alone is a carcinogen; combined estrogen and progesterone are protective against heart disease and osteoporosis.

Postmenopausal women have higher risk of osteoporosis and cardiovascular disease due to decreased estrogen.

Most common sites of endometriosis:
1. *Ovaries*
2. *Uterosacral ligament*
3. *Peritoneal surface*

Endometriosis is the most common cause of infertility in women over 30 years old with no history of PID!

OTHER CAUSES OF SECONDARY DYSMENORRHEA

Adenomyosis, ovarian cysts, pelvic adhesions, stenosis

See Table 8-2 for a discussion of adnexal masses.

TABLE 8-2 Adnexal Masses

Adnexal/ovarian masses	After detection *always* perform U/S to determine if cystic or solid!
Adnexal mass in reproductive-age woman	**Test:** U/S (cystic) ↓ Follicular or luteal cyst **Treatment:** Observation **or** **Test:** U/S (solid) ↓ Teratoma/dermoid cyst **Treatment:** Remove
Adnexal mass plus sudden onset of abdominal pain with negative B-HCG test	Torsion of ovary **Treatment:** Surgery
Adnexal mass plus pelvic/abdo pain plus fever	Tubovarian abscess
Adnexal mass plus infertility plus pain with intercourse	Perform laporoscopy Endometriosis
Adnexal mass in postmenopausal woman	Ovarian CA

Anything that decreases the number of times a woman ovulates decreases the chance for ovarian CA and vice versa.

GYN TUMORS AND CANCER

Endometrial CA = adenocarcinoma
Vulvar and cervical CA are most commonly squamous cell CA.
15% of cervical CA is adenocarcinoma.
Ovarian CA = epithelial, germ cell, or stromal
Fallopian Tube CA: Postmenopausal bleeding with **serous discharge**

BCPs are protective against endometrial CA and ovarian CA.
Pregnancy is protective against ovarian CA.
Clomiphene and HCG induce ovulation and increase risk of
ovarian CA.

Endometrial CA
Most common GYN cancer; is associated with estrogen
(carcinogen)
Presentation: Postmenopausal bleeding
Diagnostic Tests: Endometrial sampling, or if cervix
is stenosed D&C is mandatory with *any* case of
postmenopausal bleeding.
Grade is prognostic factor.
Treatment: Surgery, hormone therapy, chemo

Ovarian CA
Highest mortality of all GYN cancers
Most commonly epithelial cell but can also be germ cell or
stromal
Epithelial Ovarian CA: Serous, mucinous, Brenner
Epithelial Ovarian CA Marker: CA-125
Presentation: Most common symptom is abdominal
distension or intestinal obstruction
Treatment: Aggressive surgery and chemo
Germ Cell Ovarian Cancer: Most commonly presents in
young women
    Tumor Marker: AFP
(Stromal) Granulosa Theca Cell Tumor: Produces estrogen
and causes abnormal vaginal bleeding
(Stromal) Sertoli-Leydig Cell Tumor: Produces testosterone
and causes masculinization

Cervical CA
Most common squamous cell CA (associated with HPV)
15% adenocarcinoma
Presentation: Postcoital bleeding
Diagnostic Tests: Pelvic, speculum, Pap smear (see Figure
8-4 for follow-ups to abnormal Pap smears)
HPV 16, 18, 31, 35 related to cervical CA; HPV 6, 11 cause
genital warts, not CA
Precancerous lesions are limited to basement membrane.
Cervical CA mortality is related to uremia but is extremely
rare due to proper screening.

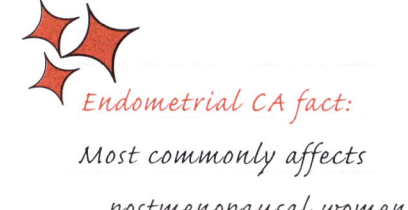

Endometrial CA fact:
Most commonly affects
postmenopausal women

Anything that increases
estrogen increases risk of
endometrial CA
#1 risk factor for endometrial
CA: Obesity

Endometrial CA fact:
Main risk factor is *obesity*
due to estrogen storage in
adipose.

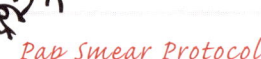

Pap Smear Protocol

Initially at 18 years old or
onset of sexual intercourse
3 successive Pap smears for 3
years
If all smears are normal,
decrease to every 2–3 years

FIGURE 8-4 Abnormal Pap Smear

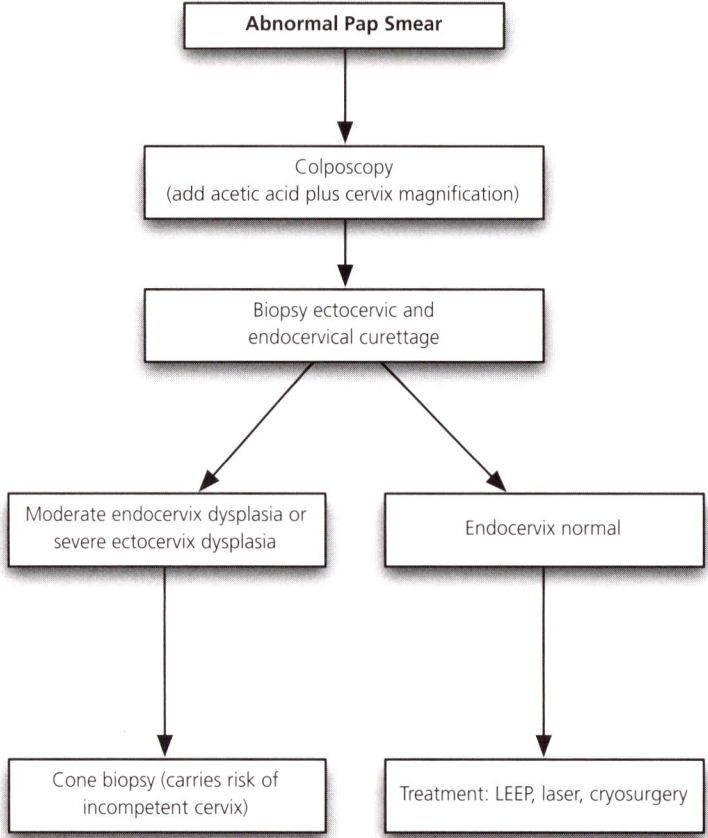

Always biopsy all vulvar
lesions.

DES is associated with:

T-shaped uterus
Columnar epithelium in
vagina

Incompetent cervix =
increased incidence of
second trimester miscarriage

Vulvar CA
Most commonly presents as itchy lesion
Most commonly squamous cell CA
Paget's Disease: Red vulvar lesion that is commonly associated with other cancers
Melanoma: Aggressive black lesion; depth of invasion is key prognostic factor

Clear Cell Adenocarcinoma of Vagina
Associated with DES exposure

INFECTIONS

See Table 8-3 for the different types of vaginitis.

TABLE 8-3 Vaginitis

Candida	Hemophilus (Gardnerella)	Trichomonas
Discharge: Sticky cottage cheese–like discharge	**Discharge:** Grayish-white and fishy	**Discharge:** Green and frothy with air bubbles
Symptom: Pruritis	**Symptom:** Odor	**Symptom:** Strawberry cervix
KOH prep = pseudohyphae	KOH = fishy odor Micro: clue cells	Motile trichomonads
pH 4	pH 5	pH 6
Treatment: Miconazole or fluconazole	**Treatment:** Metronidazole*	**Treatment:** Metronidazole*

*Metro is contraindicated in first trimester of pregnancy.

Basic evaluation for all
vaginal infections:
Vaginal pH
Wet mount and KOH prep
Gram stain
U/A

SEXUALLY TRANSMITTED DISEASES (STDS)

Chlamydia and gonorrhea are
the most common causes of
PID.

Chlamydia
Mostly asymptomatic, possible yellow-green discharge
Diagnostic Test: Gram stain reveals PMNs and *no* bacteria (PCR is best test)
Treatment: Doxycycline; if pregnant, erythromycin

Gonorrhea
Asymptomatic or yellow-green discharge
Diagnostic Tests: Gram negative diplococci, culture on Thayer-Martin agar
Treatment: Ceftrioxone, also treat for chlamydia

Syphilis
Treponema pallidum, painless, red, round chancre
Screening Test: VDRL screening; FTA is specific and diagnostic (positive for life)
Diagnostic Test: Dark-field microscopy
Treatment: IM penicillin

3 Stages of Syphilis:
1. Primary: Onset about 8 weeks—painless chancre
2. Secondary: 2 months–2 years—condyloma acuminata, rash on palms and soles
3. Tertiary: Years after onset—gummas, neurological symptoms, tabes dorsalis, Argyll-Robertson pupil, dementia

Test: VDRL or RPR confirm—FTA-ABS

Granuloma Inguinale (Donovanosis)
Painless, beefy red ulcer
Diagnostic Test: Ulcer smear = Donovani bodies
Treatment: Doxycycline

Chancroid
Painful ulcer; inguinale lymphadenopathy
Haemophilus ducreyi
Treatment: Ceftriaxone, erythromycin, or ciprofloxacin

Molluscum Contagiosum
Raised lesion with central dimple
Microscopy: Characteristic inclusion bodies
Treatment: Cryotherapy

PID
Most commonly caused by gonorrhea or chlamydia
Presentation: Adnexal mass plus abdominal pain plus fever plus leukocytosis (with or without abnormal discharge), chandelier sign (cervical motion tenderness)
Diagnostic Test: Laparoscopy
Acute PID: Commonly presents 7–10 days after menses
Treatment: Cephalosporin plus tetracycline
Chronic PID: Can cause tubovarian abscess that requires hospitalization

PID: Most common cause of infertility in normal women under 30 years old!

TOXIC SHOCK SYNDROME

Caused by staph aureus toxin (TSST-1)
Presentation: Tampon use plus fever, diarrhea, *desquamating rash*, possible shock
Treatment: IV nafcillin or oxacillin, steroids

INCONTINENCE

This is a *high yield* section for the boards.

Genuine Stress Incontinence
Symptomatic when coughs, sneezes, or laughs and *not during sleep*
Cause: Loss of pelvic floor tone/no detrusor contractions
Diagnostic: Normal neuro exam with *positive Q-tip test*
Treatment: Kegel exercises (also estrogen may improve)
Long-Term: Urethropexy

Urge Incontinence
Associated with history of sexual abuse
Cause: Involuntary detrusor contractions
Treatment: Antidepressants may improve
Long-Term: Oxybutin

Overflow Incontinence
Associated with epidural/spinal anesthetics, neuropathies, ganglionic blockers, and anticholinergics
Cause: Bladder is denervated anatomically or functionally
Diagnostic: Distended bladder with high postvoid film
Treatment: Long-term bethenachol and alpha-blockers
For spinal anesthesia, try temporary intermittent catheterization.

BIRTH CONTROL

Diaphragm
Latex over cervix
Remains in vagina 6–8 hours after intercourse
Increased risk of TSS and UTI

IUD
Small device placed in uterus
Destroys sperm
Increased risk of PID (actinomyces)
Increased risk of ectopic pregnancy

BCPs
Inhibit ovulation
Increased risk of PE, DVT
Increased risk of hepatic adenomas

Medroxyprogesterone (Depo-Provera)
Injection every 3 months
Delayed ovulation after use is stopped

"Morning-After Pill"
Estrogen plus progesterone taken within 72 hours of sexual encounter
Side Effects: Nausea and vomiting

Surgical Sterilization
Ligate tubes
Irreversible
Increased risk for ectopic pregnancy

TABLE 8-4 Infertility Evaluation and Normal Semen Criteria

Normal Semen Criteria	Infertility Evaluation (in order)
20 million/mL	1. Semen analysis
50% > forward motility	2. Document ovulation
60% > normal morphology	3. Tubal/uterine evaluation
1mL > volume	(hysterosalpingogram)

CHAPTER 9 HEMATOLOGY

ANEMIA

Hemoglobin < 14 mg/dL (males)

Hemoglobin < 12 mg/dL (females)

Presentation: Fatigue, palpitations, dyspnea on exertion, syncope, light-headedness; pallor of sclera and mucous membranes, systolic ejection murmur

Diagnosing Anemia

1. CBC with differential and RBC indices. Hemoglobin and hematocrit will be low. MCV indicates
    *   Microcytic (MCV < 80) (see Table 9-1)
    *   Normocytic (MCV 80–100)
    *   Macrocytic (MCV > 100)
2. Reticulocyte Index (RI): Measures the function of bone marrow
    *   RI < 2% = Marrow is not responding
    *   RI > 2% = Normal with anemia
3. Peripheral smear: Key findings = easy diagnosis

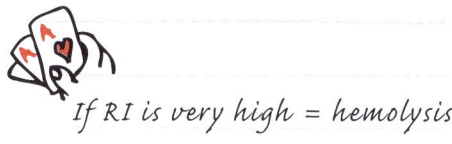

If RI is very high = hemolysis

See also Figure 9-1.

FIGURE 9-1 Anemia

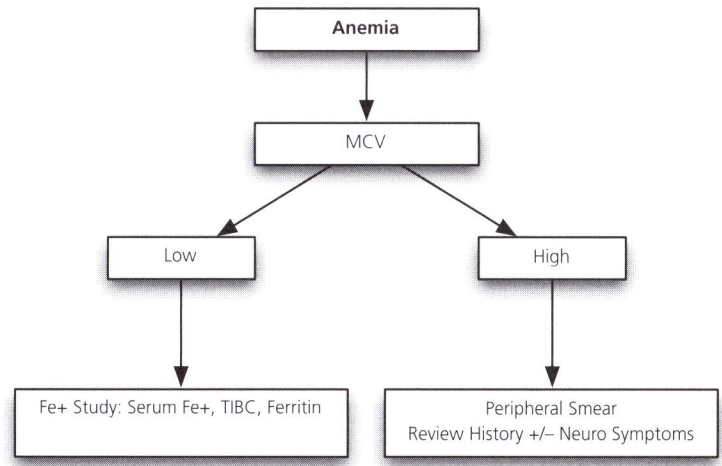

TABLE 9-1 Microcytic Anemia (MCV < 80)

	Serum Fe+	TIBC	Ferritin	Other
Fe+ Deficiency	Decreased	Increased	Decreased	> 40 years old, rule out colon CA
Chronic Disease	Decreased or Normal	Decreased	Increased	Ferritin is an acute phase reactant
Sideroblastic	Increased	Increased or Normal	Increased or Normal	Most specific test: Prussian blue stain = "ringed sideroblast" Trt: B6
Thalassemia	Normal	Normal	Normal	Hb electrophoresis

TABLE 9-2 Types of Anemia

Microcytic	Normocytic	Macrocytic
Iron Deficiency	Hemolysis	B_{12} Deficiency
Chronic Disease	Chronic Disease	Folate Deficiency
Sideroblastic	Alcohol	Thalassemia

Plummer-Vinson Syndrome
Esophageal web = glossitis and Fe+ deficiency anemia

Thalassemias

A	A2	F
Alpha2 Beta2	Alpha2 Delta2	Alpha2 Gamma2

Alpha has 4 genes; beta has 2 genes

ALPHA THALASSEMIA
Alpha chains are underproduced.
HbH: Beta4 tetramers and lacks 3 alpha globin genes
HbBarts: Gamma4 tetramers and lacks 4 alpha globin genes = hydrops fetalis

BETA THALASSEMIAS
Increased A2 and F (only seen with beta)
Beta minor: Missing 1 gene, with or without symptoms

Beta major: No beta chains; have A2 and F but no HbA
Need HbA at 6 months of age, therefore at 6 months
  of age you see symptoms of cyanosis, hypoxia,
  severe anemia requiring blood transfusion, which
  can lead to secondary hemochromatosis.
Presentation: Nucleated RBCs, target cells,
  splenomegaly, abnormal skull x-ray, plus family
  history
Diagnostic Test: Hb electrophoresis.
Treatment: Blood transfusion; iron chelating therapy
  can help prevent hemochromatosis.

Macrocytic Anemia (MCV > 100)
Smear reveals hypersegmented neutrophils and large oval
  erythrocytes with poikilocytosis

FOLATE DEFICIENCY
Most commonly seen in pregnant women and
  alcoholics.
Folate is found in green vegetables and citrus fruit.
Other Causes: Methotrexate, phenytoin, bactrim, poor
  diet (elderly eating only tea and toast)
Diagnostic Test: Folate levels
Treatment: Folate

B_{12} DEFICIENCY
Most common complaint is "pins and needles."
B_{12} is found in meat, eggs, and milk.
Presentation: Neurologic problems—motor, sensory,
  ataxia, position, vibration, cognition, psychiatric,
  autonomic
Diagnostic Tests:
  1. MCV
  2. B_{12}
To determine the specific etiology, administer
  Schilling's Test.
Causes of B_{12} Deficiency: Pernicious anemia—
  antiparietal cell antibodies and increased gastrin
  levels; *Diphyllobothrium latum* infection; terminal
  ileum resection
Treatment: B_{12}

Schilling's Test
Give radioactive B_{12}:
Decrease in urine B_{12} = lack of
  absorption
Give intrinsic factor:
If normal = pernicious anemia
If abnormal = intestinal cause

Normocytic Anemia (MCV = 80–100)

HEMOLYSIS (GENERAL)
Weakness, fatigue, dark urine, jaundice
Increased LDH, reticulocyte count, and indirect
   bilirubin

FIGURE 9-2 Coomb's Test

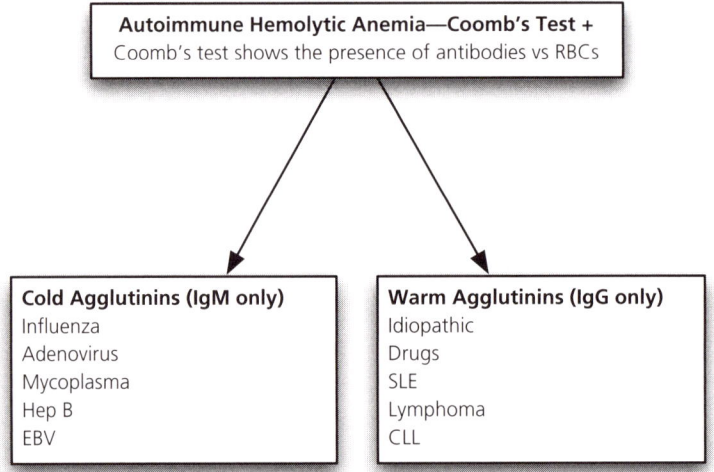

HEMOGLOBINURIA
Massive intravascular hemolysis, can cause acute
   tubular necrosis = hemosiderin in urine

TABLE 9-3 Peripheral Smear Clues of Anemia

RBC	Cause
Howell-Jolly Bodies	Asplenia: Nuclear remnant that should have been removed by the spleen
Target Cells	Thalassemia; asplenia
Teardrop RBC	Myelofibrosis: squeezed out of bone marrow
Spherocytes	Hereditary spherocytosis
Sickle Cell	Sickle cell anemia
Schistocytes	Artificial heart valve or intravascular hemolysis
Rouleaux Formation	Multiple myeloma

Fragmented RBCs	Intravascular hemolysis
Elliptocytes	Hereditary elliptocytosis
Ringed Sideroblast	Sideroblastic anemia
Heinz Bodies	G6PD
Burr Cells	ARF/Uremia
Blister Cells	G6PD
Bite Cells	Hemolytic anemia
Basophilic Stippling	Lead poisoning
Acanthocytes/Spur Cells	Abetalipoproteinemia

Glucose-6-Phosphate Dehydrogenase Deficiency

(XR) Most common in Mediterranean people

Presentation: Very sudden onset of hemolysis/anemia

Causes: Anything that causes oxidant stress

    Infection (most common)

    Fava bean ingestion

    Sulfa, dapsone, primaquine

Diagnostic Test: RBS enzyme assay

Treatment: Determine cause and discontinue it.

Sickle Cell Anemia

Almost always seen in African Americans

Presentation: No symptoms until 6 months old (time adult Hb production begins)

Dactylitis (infants)

Autosplenectomy (increased risk of encapsulated bug infections)

Pigment cholelithiasis

Bone pain (avascular necrosis of femoral head)

Salmonella osteomyelitis

Aplastic crises induced by parvovirus B19 infection

Sickle Crisis: RBC sickling causes severe pain in various sites; most common cause is infection

Crisis Treatment: Hydroxyurea (increases HbF), fluids, O_2, analgesics

Diagnostic Tests: Smear—sickled erythrocytes, Howell-Jolly bodies

Labs: High percentage of reticulocytes

Definitive Test: Hb electrophoresis

Treatment: (At time of diagnosis) folate, hydration, vaccines (plus pneumococcal), and prophylactic antibiotics

Hereditary Spherocytosis (AD)
Caused by spectrin problem in RBC membrane
Hemolysis plus large spleen
Diagnostic Tests: Increased MCHC, smear reveals spherocytes
Key: Positive osmotic fragility test
Treatment: Splenectomy

Aplastic Anemia
Pancytopenia due to lack of progenitor cells in bone marrow
Cause: AML, ALL, chemo, drugs (sulfa, AXT, chloramphenicol, carbamazepine, benzene)
Diagnostic Tests: Pancytopenia, bone marrow biopsy shows hypocellularity
Treatment: Stop causal agent

POLYCYTHEMIA VERA

Increased RBC production
Presentation: Fever, malaise, and pruritis ("itchy, especially after a warm shower")
Associated with Budd-Chiari syndrome and increased risk of leukemia
Diagnostic Tests: O_2 saturation is normal, HCT > 50, increased RBC mass, decreased erythropoietin; bone marrow biopsy shows hypercellularity
Treatment: Serial phlebotomy, daily aspirin

FIGURE 9-3 Erythropoietin Levels

PRV: ⬇ Erythropoietin
Secondary polycythemia due to hypoxia (COPD, etc.):
⬆ Erythropoietin
Absence of hypoxia, ⬆ Erythropoietin: renal cell carcinoma

PAROXYSMAL HEMOGLOBINURIA

pH change caused by CO_2 retention at night
Presentation: Dark morning urine and major venous thrombosis (ex. portal vein)
Diagnostic Tests: Sugar water and Hamm's test (Key: These tests are unique to PNH.)
Treatment: Steroids

IDIOPATHIC THROMBOCYTOPENIA PURPURA

Autoimmune in origin
May follow viral illness in children; adult form is chronic.
Most common in sixth decade and affects females to males
    2:1.
Afebrile, no splenomegaly, petechiae and purpura
Diagnostic Tests: Low platelets, possible anemia
Key: Positive platelets associated with IgG
Treatment: Mild: steroids, moderate platelets
        Severe: IVIG and Rho(D) (Rh+ patients)
        Chronic: splenectomy

HEMOLYTIC UREMIC SYNDROME

Seen with *E. coli* 0157: H7 food poisoning
Hemolysis uremia thrombocytopenia syndrome (HUS)
Diagnostic Tests: No specific test, PT/PTT are normal
Treatment: Usually spontaneous resolution; if life
    threatening—plasmapheresis

THROMBOTIC THROMBOCYTOPENIA PURPURA

HUS plus fever, altered mental status, splenomegaly
Diagnostic Tests: High bleeding time, low platelets and
    RBCs, normal PT/PTT
Treatment: Plasmapheresis

Do not give platelets to TTP patients!

DISSEMINATED INTRAVASCULAR COAGULATION

Commonly seen in: Pregnancy/obstetric complications,
    malignancy, sepsis, trauma
Presentation: Oozing/bleeding from puncture sites
Diagnostic Tests: Increased bleeding time, D-dimers, fibrin-
    split product; decreased fibrinogen
Treatment: Cryoprecipitate and platelets

FIGURE 9-4 DIC, TIP, HUS, and PT/PTT

DIC activates clotting cascade = ⬆ PT/PTT
TTP and HUS affect aggregation of platelets and PT/PTT
    are normal.

HEMOPHILIA

X-linked recessive
Factor VIII—Hemophilia A
Factor IX—Hemophilia B
Presentation: Boy with excessive bleeding or hemarthrosis after mild trauma
Diagnostic Test: Increased PTT
Treatment: Factor VIII or Factor IX: desmopressin—use as prophylaxis before minor medical procedures

VON WILLEBRAND'S DISEASE

Autosomal dominant
Most common inherited blood disorder
Factor VIII deficiency plus decreased platelet adhesions
Presentation: Easy bleeding, easy bruising, epistaxis, and heavy menstrual bleeding
Aspirin exacerbates condition
Diagnostic Tests: PTT normal or increased, increased BT, decreased ristocetin
Ristocetin: Measures the ability to agglutinate platelets by vWF
Treatment: Mild—desmopressin; major—cryoprecipitate or FFP; BCPs for women of reproductive age

FACTOR V LEIDEN

Most common hereditary cause of hypercoagulable state. Factor V mutation decreases the activation of Protein C. Predisposes patients to CVAs, PEs, DVTs.

TRANSFUSIONS

Whole blood: Used for blood loss
Packed RBCs: Most common type of transfusion; used instead of whole blood
Washed RBCs: Given to patients with IgA deficiency and allergic patients
Platelets: Given when platelets > 10,000/microL
Cryoprecipitate: Has Factor VIII and fibrinogen (trt. of DIC and vWF)
Fresh Frozen Plasma: Has all clotting factors (trt. of DIC or warfarin poisoning); used when you cannot wait for vitamin K to take effect

Blood Transfusion Reaction

Due to preformed recipient antibodies that cause acute
hemolysis during RBC transfusions.

Suspect transfusion reaction? When determining cause
always think of the following:

1. Most common cause is clerical error.
2. IgA deficiency patients who are sensitized are at
   risk for anaphylaxis.

Presentation: Shortly after transfusion is started,
anxiety, pain, hypotension, tachycardia, fever, chills,
hemoglobinuria.

Hemoglobinuria: Hb released with massive hemolysis can
cause acute tubular necrosis.

Diagnostic Tests: Stop transfusion and double-check
patient's blood type; test for free Hb in urine and blood;
labs to rule out DIC.

Treatment: Discontinue transfusion; give IV fluids, mannitol
(to help prevent oliguria).

*Blood transfusion reaction:
Most commonly caused by
clerical error!*

*In emergency situation or if
you do not know patient's
blood type give Type O
Negative blood.*

ONCOLOGY

In children and young adults, leukemia is the most common
cancer, but *age* is a major factor that increases the
incidence and mortality of cancer.

Leukemia

Most leukemias are B-cell in origin.

The elevated cell line is leukemic; all other cell lines are
depressed.

Acute—starts in bone marrow

Chronic—starts in periphery

ALL

Age: 1–5 years old; peak age: 3–5 years old

80% of all childhood leukemias

Presentation: Bone pain, easy bruising, fever,
petechia/purpura, bleeding, hepatosplenomegaly

Labs: Neutropenia, anemia, thrombocytopenia
Increased LDH and uric acid
Bone marrow biopsy = increased lymphoblasts
TdT +
CALLA + (marker for good prognosis)

Treatment: Chemotherapy causes remission in 85% of
childhood patients.

AML

Age: Over 30 years old

Types:

M3—DIC

M5—gingival hyperplasia

Presentation: Frequent infection, easy bruising, anemia, dyspnea, fatigue, fever, petechiae/purpura

Labs: Pancytopenia; may see increased myeloblasts (neutros, basos, eos, erythros, megakaryos); stain with Sudan black

Diagnostics:

- Auer rods
- Myeloperoxidase
- Decreased LAP score

AML Types:

M1—No differentiation; myeloblasts

M2—Differentiation; myeloblasts, promyeloblasts

M3—Auer rods; promyelocytes

M5—Positive for nonspecific esterase; promonocytes

M7—React with antiplatelet antibodies; megakaryocytes

Treatment: Chemotherapy and bone marrow transplant; retinoic acid for AML-M3 type

CML

Age: 30–50 years old.

Cells are more mature vs AML; presents in periphery with less bone marrow involvement

CML often stable for many years until *blast crisis*, which converts it to AML

Presentation: Fever, fatigue, malaise, weight loss, night sweats

Labs: WBC > 50,000, *massive* splenomegaly

Definitive Diagnosis: Philadelphia chromosome (9:22)

Treatment: Poor prognosis; (chronic) alpha interferon and hydroxyurea; allogenic BMT curative in about 60% of cases

CLL

Seen in patients older than 55

Can live for many years without treatment

Mature B-cell problem with no bone marrow involvement

Presentation: Diffuse lymphadenopathy
Labs: Lymphocytosis only
Diagnostic: CD5+; smudge cells
Treatment: Supportive; chemo for exacerbations

HAIRY CELL LEUKEMIA
50-year-old man with a big, hard spleen
Blood Smear: Hairy cells and TRAP +

NON-HODGKINS LYMPHOMA
Any age
Small Follicular Type: Most common and best prognosis
Large Diffuse Type: Worst prognosis
CNS B-Cell Lymphoma: Look for HIV+/AIDS
Burkitt's Lymphoma: Caused by Epstein-Barr virus (EBV)
- Mostly affects children
- U.S.—abdomen
- Africa—Jaw

Mutation: C-myc Bcl-2
Tumor Lysis Syndrome: Seen in high grade NHL and is due to rapid tumor cell death
Labs: Decreased Ca+ and increased Phosphate, Uric Acid, Potassium
For Hodgkin's vs non-Hodgkin's lymphoma, see Figure 9-5.

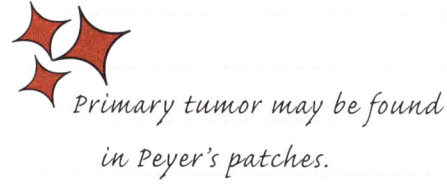
Primary tumor may be found in Peyer's patches.

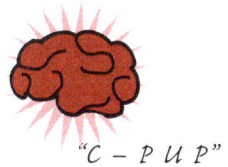
"C – P U P"

FIGURE 9-5 Hodgkin's vs Non-Hodgkin's Lymphoma

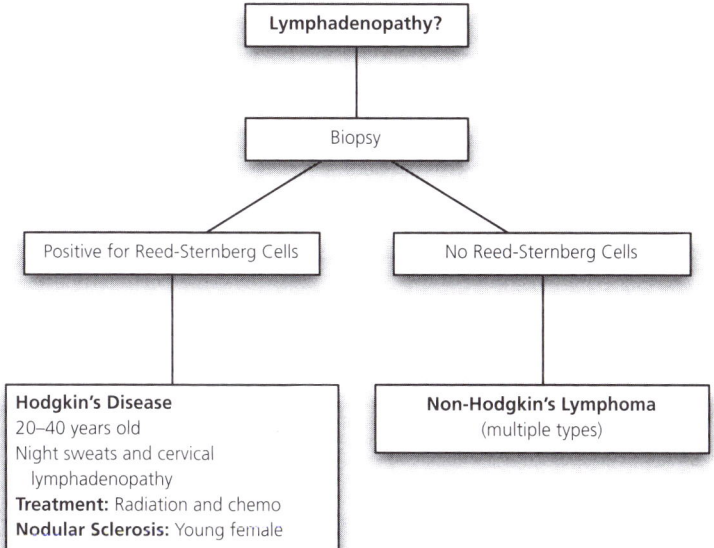

MM is an osteoclastic problem; therefore use x-ray not bone scan. Bone scan only shows osteoblastic problems.

MULTIPLE MYELOMA

Age: Over 50 years old

Malignant expansion of plasma cells and excessive production of Igs (50% IgG, 25% IgA)

Presentation: Hypercalcemia symptoms (bones, stones, and psychiatric overtones), bone/back pain, kidney stones, psych symptoms

Tests: Serum/urine protein electrophoresis—monoclonal gammopathy (IgG)

Diagnostic: Bence-Jones proteinuria and punched-out lesions on skull/long bone x-ray

Treatment: Chemo, steroids

WALDENSTROM'S DISEASE

Age: Over 40 years old

A "hyperviscosity" syndrome

Presentation: Raynaud's with cold insensitivity

Tests: IgM spike, cold agglutinins

PRIMARY THROMBOCYTOPENIA

Age: Over 50 years old

Presentation: Bleeding or thrombosis

Diagnostic: > 1,000,000 platelet count

T-CELL LEUKEMIA

Caused by HTLV-1

MYCOSIS FUNGOIDES (RASH)/SÉZARY SYNDROME (BLOOD)

Age: Over 50 years old

T-cell in origin

Presentation: Plaquelike, itchy skin rash with Pautrier abscesses = leonine facies

Complication: Can transform into lymphoma

Blood Smear: Cerebriform nuclei, butt cells

Treatment: PUVA chemo, steroids

CHAPTER 10 INFECTIOUS DISEASE

VAGINITIS

See Table 8-3 in Chapter 8 for more information on vaginitis.

STDS

See Chapter 8 for information on chlamydia, gonorrhea, syphilis, granuloma inguinale (donovanosis), chancroid, molluscum contagiosum, PID, and toxic shock syndrome.

HSV 1 or 2
Painful, itchy, multiple red shallow vesicles
Diagnostic Test: Tzanck smear or viral culture
Treatment: Acyclovir for breakouts

HPV
Painless, itchy warts (pink cauliflower-like)
Condyloma acuminata—serotypes 6 and 11
Diagnostic Tests: Clinical exam, biopsy
Treatment: Topical—trichloracetic acid, podophyllin; cryotherapy
HPV 16, 18, 31, 35 associated with cervical CA

UTI

Most commonly affects women
E. coli (most common), *S. saprophyticus*, Proteus, pseudomonas, serratia, Enterobacter
Risk Factors: Foley catheter, BPH, reflux, history of previous UTIs or pylenophritis, DM, immunosuppresion, pregnancy
Presentation: Increased urinary frequency, urgency, and pain
Diagnostic Tests: Urine dipstick—increased nitrites, leukocyte esterase, hematuria (cystitis), urine pH (proteus); WBC casts: pylenophritis; microscopic: > 5 RBC per high power field
Gold Standard: > 10^5 bacteria per mL
Treatment: TMP-SMX or ciprofloxacin

Basic evaluation for all vaginal infections:
Vaginal pH
Wet mount and KOH prep
Gram stain
U/A

PYLENOPHRITIS

Presentation: UTI symptoms plus fever and costovertebral angle tenderness

Diagnostic Tests: Urinalysis—WBC casts; CBC—leukocytosis

Treatment: Fluids, antibiotics 3 days inpatient, then about 2.5 weeks outpatient

See Figure 10-1 for examples of when further evaluation is needed in pylenophritis patients.

FIGURE 10-1 Further Evaluation of Pylenophritis

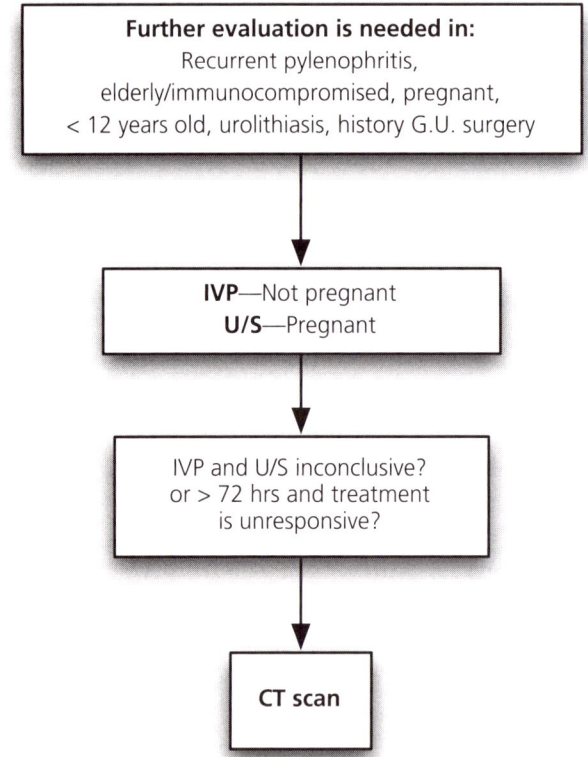

Further evaluation is needed in:
Recurrent pylenophritis,
elderly/immunocompromised, pregnant,
< 12 years old, urolithiasis, history G.U. surgery

IVP—Not pregnant
U/S—Pregnant

IVP and U/S inconclusive?
or > 72 hrs and treatment
is unresponsive?

CT scan

STREP PYOGENES (A)

Poststreptococcal glomerulonephritis: Most commonly after strep skin infection

Pharyngitis: Positive strep test; treat to avoid scarlet fever

Rheumatic Fever: Sore throat followed by two Jones criteria

Scarlet Fever: Erythrogenic toxin; strawberry tongue; truncal red, blotchy rash

Rheumatic Fever

Cause is untreated strep throat; therefore look for previous sore throat in question stem.

Most commonly affects mitral valve (onset 2 weeks after sore throat).

Must have two or more from list of Jones criteria for diagnosis:

- Subcutaneous nodules
- Polyarthritis
- Erythema marginatum
- Chorea
- Carditis

Only Strep Throat = Rheumatic Fever

Strep Throat or Skin Strep can = Poststrep glomerulonephritis

ENDOCARDITIS

Mitral valve most commonly affected

Risk: Congenital heart disease, valvular disease, prosthetic heart valves, IVDU

Strep bovis—GI malignancy

Candida/Aspergillus (fungal)—immunosuppression

Presentation: New onset heart murmur, fever, Osler's nodes, splinter hemorrhage, Janeway lesions, Roth spots

Diagnostic Test: Duke's criteria

Confirmative: Positive blood cultures (two at two different times/sites) plus echo

Treatment: IV antibiotics, vancomycin or ceftriaxone and gentamycin

If undergoing surgery, offer prophylaxis to susceptible patients: IVDU, valvular disease, congenital heart defects.

Subacute Bacterial Endocarditis vs Acute Bacterial Endocarditis

Strep Viridans—Left side (Mitral)

Staph Aureus—Right side (IVDU)

AIRWAY

Croup

Parainfluenza virus

Peak Age: 4–5 years old, usually in winter

Presentation: Inspiratory stridor, barking cough

Diagnostic Test: X-ray shows steeple sign

Treatment: Steroids and humidified air

Epiglottitis

H. influenza

Peak Age: 3–10 years old

Presentation: Muffled voice, leaning forward and drooling, cherry red epiglottis

Treatment: Emergency; take to OR and intubate immediately

Test: Thumbprint sign on x-ray, but if you suspect this illness, don't wait for x-ray results to take action

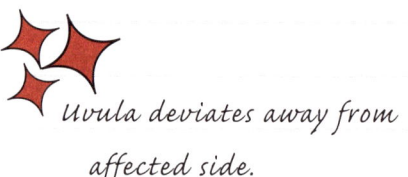

Uvula deviates away from

affected side.

Pharyngitis
Group A strep
Diagnostic Test: Throat culture
Complications: GN, rheumatic fever

Retropharyngeal Abscess
High fever, drooling
Diagnostic Test: Lateral x-ray

Peritonsilar Abscess
High fever, bulging swollen tonsils, "hot potato voice"
Treatment: Culture abscess

Aspiration Pneumonia
Common in patients with neurological disorders
"Foreign body" aspiration pneumonia: common in
   pediatrics (right middle or lower lobe)

Pneumonia
Differentiate between typical and atypical bugs; see Table
   10-1.
Diagnostic Tests: Elevated WBCs and CXR abnormalities
Confirmatory Tests: Sputum culture and blood culture

For pneumonia key words, see Table 10-2.

TABLE 10-1 Pneumonia

	Atypical Pneumonia	Typical Pneumonia
Age	< 45 years old	> 45 years old
Fever	< 102 degrees	> 102 degrees
Prodrome	> 3 days	< 2 days
CXR	Single lobe	Diffuse
Bug	Mycoplasma, chlamydia, etc.	Strep pneumoniae
Medications	Azithromycin	Cephalosporins

TABLE 10-2 Pneumonia Key Words

Pneumonia in cystic fibrosis	*Pseudomonas*
Lung abscess after pneumonia	*Staph aureus*
Pneumonia in bird handler	*Chlamydia psittaci*
(Rods) In homeless and alcoholics; "currant jelly sputum"	*Klebsiella*
Aspiration, hospital acquired, neutropenia	*E. coli*
College student (atypical)	Mycoplasma
Silver stain	*P. carinii,* legionella, mycoplasma
Lung fungus ball 45-degree v-shaped hyphae	*Aspergillus fumigatus*

CAUSES

Typical
Staphylococcus Aureus: Gram positive cocci in clusters
IVDU, hospital acquired
Key: Recurrent lung abscesses; empyema
Streptococcus Pneumoniae: Gram positive diplococci
Common in elderly
Fever, productive cough
Key: Rust-colored sputum
Diagnostic Tests: X-ray—lobar consolidation; high neutrophils
Treatment: Third-gen cephalosporin or azithromycin
Hemophilus Influenza: Gram negative coccobacilli
More common in kids
Treatment: Second-, third-gen cephalosporin, ampicillin/amoxicillin

Atypical
Mycoplasma: Young adults
Diagnostic Test: Positive cold agglutinin
Treatment: Azithromycin
Legionella: Hotel air-conditioning (water source)
Diagnostic Test: Silver stain
Treatment: Erythromycin

Blast-o, Coccidi-o, Paracoccidi-o,

Histo-

- *Culture on Sabouraud*
- *Turns to yeast in tissue*
- *Systemic treatment—Ampho B*
- *Local treatment—-azole*

Histoplasmosis
Histoplasma capsulatum

Endemic: Cave dwelling in Ohio, Mississippi

Presentation: Flulike symptoms with or without erythema nodosum or erythema multiforme

Risk Factors: Cave dwelling, bird droppings, HIV infection

Diagnostic Tests: Quick diag—complement fixation Ab's; silver stain on biopsy or bronchoalveolar lavage

Treatment: Ketoconazole, ampho B; HIV +—IV amphotericin B and lifelong itraconazole

Coccidioidomycosis
Coccidioides immitus

Endemic: Southwest United States (San Joaquin Valley)

Presentation: Flulike symptoms of pneumonia and possible desert bumps

Diagnostic Tests: Serology; IgM rise 2 wks–2 months; IgG 1–3 months

Treatment: Ampho B, -azoles

Blastomycosis
Big, broad-based budding

Endemic: Mississppi River and Central America

Paracoccidiomycosis
Endemic: Latin America

"Captain's wheel" appearance

Cryptococcus
Cryptococcus neoformans

Found in pigeon droppings

"AIDS-defining illness": Almost exclusively seen in immunocompromised patients

Presentation: Pneumonia-like symptoms followed by meningitis

Diagnostic Tests: LP—low glucose, high protein, high lymphocytes; positive India ink of CSF

Treatment: Ampho B

HIV

Retrovirus

Risk Factors: Unprotected sex, IVDU

Extent of disease: CD 4 count; rate of disease progression: viral load

Presentation:
> Initially—possible asymptomatic, flulike symptoms, lymphadenopathy
> Later—symptoms related to immunosuppression

Diagnostic Test: ELISA
Confirmatory: Western blot
Treatment: CD 4 < 500 protease inhibitors—-ivir; nonnucleoside reverse transcriptase inhibitors; two nucleoside analogs AZT, ddI, 3tc, D4T

Ways to Decrease HIV Transmission to Babies

Pregnant HIV patients—treat mother with AZT and give AZT to baby for 6 weeks after birth.

C-section reduces vertical transmission.

Breast-feeding is contraindicated in HIV+ mothers.

Due to mom's Abs baby will have false positive for 6–12 months.

Confirmatory diagnostic test for baby 6–12 months old is PCR (directly detects virus).

CMV

Intracellular inclusion bodies treatment: gancyclovir, alternate foscarnet

Cryptosporidium

Diarrhea unique to HIV patients

CD 4 Counts and Prophylaxis

PNEUMOCYSTIC CARINII (PCP)

CD < 200, silver stain
Treatment: TMX-SFM alternate: pentamidine

MYCOBACTERIUM AVIUM INTRACELLULAR (MAI)

CD 4 < 100
Treatment: Clarithromycin alternate: azithromycin, rifabutin

Administer: Annual pneumococcus and influenza vaccine
Can also receive MMR (only live), SALK, Hep B
> Annual PPD, CXR

HIV diagnosis: CD4 (2 times per year)

Begin drug treatment: CD 4 < 500

AIDS diagnosis: CD 4 < 200

Watch out for AIDS cancers: Kaposi's sarcoma and non-Hodgkin's.

PPD: proves previous exposure, not active infection

Positive test determined by size of induration (read 2–3 days after injection):

> 5 mm: HIV

>10 mm: homeless, immigrant, crowded living conditions

> 15 mm: normal health

TUBERCULOSIS

Mycobacterium tuberculosis
Symptomatic cases due to reactivation of old infection
Risk Factors: Alcohol, immunosuppression, DM, homeless, crowded living conditions, health care workers and others with high sick contacts, immigrants from developing countries
Presentation: Fever, weight loss, night sweats, cough, hemoptysis
Diagnostic Test: Positive sputum acid-fast stain (results take weeks)
Confirmed Diagnosis: Positive PPD, suspicious CXR, positive sputum culture

CXR

Nodular infiltrates with or without cavitation
Treatment: INH (plus vitamin B_6), rifampin (body fluid discoloration); pyrazinamide; ethambutol; streptomycin
Pregnant: avoid streptomycin; it is teratogenic.

ANTHRAX

Bacillus anthracis G+ spore former
People who handle animal wool and animal products (farmers, veterinarians, herders)
3 Types:
- Cutaneous (most common)
- Inhalation (most severe)
- Intestinal

Presentation for Cutaneous:
1. Pruritic papule erupts a few days after exposure.
2. 1–2 days papule grows to ulcer.
3. 1 week ulcer turns into **black eschar** with edema.

Diagnostic Test: Aerobic/G stain reveals nonmotile bacilli chains
Treatment: Penicillin plus 2 months ciprofloxacin to prevent inhalation type

OSTEOMYELITIS

Fever and localized bone pain
Direct spread or via bloodstream
Causes: See Table 10-3.
Diagnostic Tests: MRI, indium-labeled leukocyte scan, bone aspiration
Treatment: IV antibiotics and debridement

TABLE 10-3 Causes of Osteomyelitis

Bug	Key Hints
Pseudomonas	IVDU Puncture wound
S. epidermidis	Ortho surgery
Salmonella	Sickle cell anemia

MARJOLIN'S ULCER (SCC)

Associated with nonhealing ulcer in burn victims

OTITIS

For details of otitis, see Table 10-4.

TABLE 10-4 Otitis

	S&S	Key Hints	Treatment
Otitis Media *S. pneumoniae* *H. influenza*	Bulging tympanic membranes, landmarks difficult to visualize	No pain on manipulation	Amoxicillin
Otitis Externa *Pseudomonas*	Pain and discharge from canal in child who **swims**	Pain on manipulation, history of swimming	Polymyxin B drops

Infectious Myringitis
Mycoplasma, strep pneumo, virus
Presentation: Vesicles on tympanic membrane

VIRUSES

See Table 10-5 for a list of viral illnesses.

TABLE 10-5 Viral Illnesses

Disease	Cause	Key
Fifth's Disease, Erythema Infectiosum	Parvovirus B19	"Slapped cheek" appearance—may cause aplastic anemia.
Measles	Rubeola—possible complication is SSPE	Rubeola has 4 syllables—and causes symptoms with 4 hard "ck" sounds: Cough, Coryza, Conjunctivitis, Koplik spots.
3-Day Measles	Rubella	Rubella has 3 syllables—and causes 3-day measles plus lymphadenopathies.
Roseola Infantum	HHV-6—possible complication: febrile seizure	Fever 104–105°, then rash outbreak.
Mumps	Mumps—possible complication: orchitis	Parotid swelling, increased amylase.
Shingles	VZV	Vesicular rash in dermatome distribution.
Infectious Mononucleosis	EBV—Mono patient plus ampicillin = bad rash	Adolescent with flulike symptoms for 4–6 weeks—enlarged spleen CBC: atypical lymphocytes Monospot test.

DIARRHEA

Viral
Rotavirus: The most common cause of diarrhea in children
Test: Immunoassay
Treatment: Supportive

Protozoa
Treatment for all three types of protozoan diarrhea is
    metronidazole; see Table 10-6 for descriptions of the
    three types.

TABLE 10-6 Protozoa

Giardia lamblia	Causes **watery** diarrhea with abdominal distension and weight loss Caused by cyst ingestion from contaminated food or water —Commonly seen with drinking stream or well water while camping —Steathorrhea plus protozoal cysts in stool **Tests:** (Diagnostic) duodenal aspirate
Entamoeba histolytica	Causes **bloody** diarrhea and affects the colon —May have a long incubation period of up to 3 months —May mimic inflammatory bowel disease **Tests:** Stool culture, serology, biopsy
Clostridium difficile	Only seen after prior antibiotic use Example: Child plus infection plus antibiotic therapy plus diarrhea = clostridium **Tests:** *C. diff* toxin in stool (*cytotoxin assay*) Flexible sigmoidoscopy shows pseudomembranes

Cryptosporidium can also cause diarrhea, but this is almost
    exclusively seen in the immunocompromised.

*Always test for HIV in patients
    with cryptosporidium.*

Bacterial

For all bacterial causes, you will see fecal RBCs and WBCs; therefore this is not diagnostic. Pay attention to other clues in the question. See Table 10-7 for the types of bacterial diarrhea.

TABLE 10-7 Types of Bacterial Diarrhea

Campylobacter	Most common cause of infectious diarrhea —Spread via contaminated food or water Example: Ulcerative colitis–like symptoms plus arthritis = *Campylobacter* **Treatment:** Supportive, self-limited
Yersinia	Transmitted by contaminated food or animals Example: Child with acute onset RLQ pain (like appendicitis) plus diarrhea = *Yersinia* **Tests:** (Diagnostic) serology or stool culture
Shigella	Extremely contagious, person-to-person spread or from foods —Usually seen in **institutionalized patients** or **daycare centers** —Commonly causes febrile seizures in young children Example: Daycare outbreak plus child with diarrhea plus new onset seizure = *Shigella* **Treatment:** TMP-SMX
Salmonella	Spread through poultry, eggs, and milk —Associated headache, fever, malaise **Treatment:** Supportive **Antibiotics will prolong carrier state.**
Enterotoxigenic *E. coli*	"Traveler's diarrhea" —Very watery diarrhea with no blood or fever **Treatment:** TMP-SMX and loperamide
Enterohemorrhagic *E. coli:* (0157:H7)	This causes diarrhea and HUS. Example: Child with diarrhea later develops hemolysis, uremia, thrombocytopenia **Treatment:** Supportive

CSF INFECTIONS AND FINDINGS

Bacterial: Increased PMNs, decreased glucose, increased protein

Viral: Increased monos, normal glucose, normal or increased protein

Fungal: Increased monos, decreased glucose, normal or increased protein

Clues:

> India ink stain for *Cryptococcus*
>
> Giemsa stain for trypanosomes
>
> PCR for *Herpes*
>
> RBCs may be seen with HSV encephalitis
>
> CMV encephalitis treatment: gancyclovir and foscarnet

Treatment: HSV IV acyclovir

> Before culture comes back, if you suspect bacterial, give vancomycin.
>
> Close contacts for meningococcus is rifampin (side effect: turns secretions orange).

Meningococcus always causes petechiae; therefore look for it in the presentation.

TABLE 10-8 Meningitis

Less than 1 month old	Group B strep, *E. coli*, *Listeria* (G-E-L)
1–3 months	Pneumococci, Meningococci
3 months–adult	Pneumococci, Meningococci
Military/dormitory	Meningococci (*petechiae*)
Over 60 years old	Pneuomococci, G- bacilli, Listeria

Encephalitis presents the same way as meningitis but is more commonly caused by HSV, arbovirus, or pneumococcus.

SPECIFIC PRESENTATIONS

Encephalitis: *Confused*

Meningitis: Stiff neck plus photophobia

Abscess alone: Focal deficit

In general, CNS infections may present as: fever, headache, nuchal rigidity.

Upon examination: Positive Kernig's, positive Brudzinski's

> Focal neurological signs are possible.
>
> Increased ICP (papilledema).
>
> Bulging fontanelle in babies.
>
> Altered mental status.

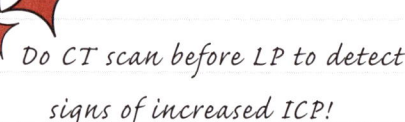

Do CT scan before LP to detect signs of increased ICP!

Use "ToRCHeS" to remember diseases/infections that can be transmitted to babies by their mothers; see Table 10-9.

Mothers with SLE will have babies with congenital heart block.

Tests:

CT may show focal lesion.
If you need CT before LP, give patient ceftriaxone.
Culture is the best, most accurate, specific, etc.

INFECTIONS PASSED FROM MOTHER TO BABY

TABLE 10-9 ToRCHeS

Disease	Cause	Key	Treatment
Toxoplasmosis First trimester is severe vs third trimester	Eating raw cat meat or changing litter box while pregnant	Intracranial calcifications, chorioretinitis **CT—Ring-enhancing lesions	Pyrimethamine, sulfadiazine, spiramycin (all for the mother)
Rubella	Transmission in first trimester	PDA, cataracts, mental retardation, hearing loss, **Blueberry muffin rash	Prevented by immunizing *before* pregnancy
CMV	Transplacentally transmitted	**Periventricular calcifications plus petechial rash	Gancylcovir
Herpes	Mom plus active lesions = intrapartum transmission	Dangerous CNS infection, skin/mouth infection	Prevent via C-section if lesions present Treatment: Acyclovir
Syphilis	Intrapartum transmission	Hepatomegaly, *snuffles*, skin rash, saber shins, Hutchinson's teeth, hearing loss	Prevented via penicillin in pregnant women

LYME DISEASE

Borrelia burgdorferi (spirochete)
Vector: Ixodes tick
MC northeast
Presentation: Rash, fever, malaise, fatigue, HA, joint/muscle pain
Primary: Erythema migrans, small red macule found at feeding site; bullseye rash
Secondary: Migratory polyarthropathies, Bell's palsy, myocarditis
Tertiary: Arthritis, mood change, memory loss
Diagnostic Tests: ELISA (exposure); Western blot (confirmatory)
Treatment: Acute—doxycycline, later ceftriaxone

ROCKY MOUNTAIN SPOTTED FEVER

Rickettsia rickettsii
Vector: Dermancentor tick (usually East Coast)
Presentation: HA, fever (around 4 days) then **rash appears**—begins on palms and soles, then changes to more purpuric as it moves centrally
Diagnostic Test: Weil-Felix test
Treatment: Doxycycline

RABIES

Bats, skunks, raccoons, or foxes, not rabbits, squirrels, chipmunks, or rodents
Vaccine has stopped dog rabies
Incubation of 1–2 months
Presentation: Hydrophobia and paralysis
Treatment: Initial bite—clean with soap and water; do not close wound
    Observe animal for rabies S&S; if wild, kill and examine tissue
    Wild animal—give prophylaxis and vaccine
    Domestic animal—No symptoms after observation do not give prophylaxis or vaccine

LOFGREN'S SYNDROME

Sarcoidosis with arthritis, ankle edema, erythema nodosum, hilar lymphadenopathy

ANTIBIOTICS AND ANTIVIRALS

Herpes/varicella: Acyclovir
CMV: Gancyclovir, foscarnet
Influenza: Oseltamivir, zanamivir
Hep B: Lamuvidine or interferon
Hep C: Interferon and ribavirin
Fungal Infection: Amphotericin B (risk of renal failure)
Candida: -azoles

Gram – Bacilli: *Klebsiella, Enterobactor, Pseudomonas, Morganella, Proteus, E. coli*
Aminoglycosides (-mycin), Quinolones (-floxiacin)

Gram + Cocci (Staph and Strep): Penicillins, -cillins
    Mild penicillin allergy—first-generation cephalosporin
    Severe penicillin allergy—macrolides or clindamycin
    Anaphylaxis to penicillin—vancomycin
Hbs AG + Acute and chronic disease
Hbs Ab + Complete recovery
Hbc Ab + Acute and window phase, complete recovery, chronic carrier
HbE—low transmissibility
Hbc Ab- + during window period

IgM Ab (HAV) Hep A is an acute infection only; therefore IgM is the best test for Hep A infection.

See Table 10-10 for a list of infectious disease key words. (Key words for pneumonia are in Table 10-2.)

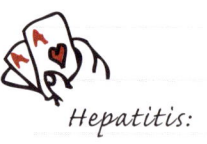

Hepatitis:

s- surface	*Ab- Antibody*
c- core	*AG- Antigen*

TABLE 10-10 Infectious Disease Key Words

CMV encephalitis	Treat with ganciclovir and foscarnet
HSV encephalitis	RBCs in CSF
Chalizion	(Granulomatous inflammation) Hard, painful lid nodule
Hordeolum	(Staph) Painful swelling of eyelid
Screen for HCV	Blood transfusion before 1992
Screen for HBV	Blood transfusion before 1986
PID with *high* fever	Hospitalize with doxycycline plus cefotetan
Chlamydia	G-stain = PMNs with no bacteria
Candida	Thrush in immunocompromised
Mucor/Rhizor	Fungus that disrupts blood vessels in DM patients
Impetigo	Honey-crusted lesions
Babeosis	Patient with jaundice, splenectomized, and from Northeast
Francisella tularensis	Tularemia; rabbit/deer bite
Yersinia pestis	Plague; fleabite from rat
Brucella	Fever plus meat handler
E. faecalis	Endocarditis, UTI, or sepsis Grow on 6.5 NaCl
Strep mutans	Dental caries
Strep viridans	Subacute bacterial endocarditis
Nesseria meningitis	Give rifampin prophylaxis to sick contacts
Pasteurella multocida	Cat/dog bite
Sporotrix schenckii	Stuck with rose thorn Treat: ketocanozole, K+ iodide
C. botulinum	Baby with paralysis after eats honey
Actinomyces israelii	Sulfur granules/branching rods PID after IUD use
Clostridium perfringens	Burn victim or gangrene
Pseudomonas	Burn infection
Spirochete	"BLT"—Borrelia, Leptospira, Treponema
Cryptococcus	Positive India ink

CHAPTER 11 MUSCULOSKELETAL

LOW BACK PAIN

Common problem; many causes
Diagnostic Tests: Primarily clinical but *always* order an x-ray
Treatment: NSAIDs, bed rest < 3 days (most recover in 6 weeks)

Most common cause is sprain or strain.

HERNIATED DISC

Most common in L4–L5, L5–S1 and commonly follows strenuous activity
Presentation: Months of aching LBP followed by sudden onset of severe LBP plus sciatica
Sciatica—pain radiating down leg exacerbated by coughing or valsalva
Diagnostic Tests: Increased pain on crossed and passive straight leg raise
Gold Standard Test: MRI
Treatment: NSAIDs, bed rest, PT; long-term symptoms, treat with discectomy

LBP x-rays may reveal:
Vertebral Lytic Lesions—
  Breast or Lung CA
Blastic Lesions—Prostate CA
Bamboo Spine—Osgood-
  Schlatter

Remember BLT with a KP METS to bone (breast, lung, thyroid, kidney, prostate).

SPINAL STENOSIS

Narrowing of lumbar or c-spine canal due to degenerative joint disease
Most commonly seen in middle-aged and elderly
Presentation: Back or neck pain with or without radiation; leg cramps may occur with walking, standing, or rest
Key Presentation: Sitting = relief
Diagnostic Tests: X-ray may show degenerative changes; CT or MRI will show stenosis.
Treatment: NSAIDs; if severe, epidural steroids

MRI is the best test.

OSGOOD-SCHLATTER

Male 10–25 years old with LBP worse in the morning plus family history (HLA-B27)
Presentation: Intermittent hip and LBP and stiffness, worse in morning
Diagnostic Test: HLA-B27
Key: X-ray reveals "bamboo spine"
Treatment: NSAIDs plus exercise

May be associated with third-degree heart block.

COMPARTMENT SYNDROME

Elevated pressure in a confined space; usually caused by injury, fracture, etc.

Presentation: Pain (out of proportion of physical findings), pallor, poikilothermia, parasthesias, paralysis, pulselessness (last two Ps seen late)

Diagnostic Tests: Primarily clinical; otherwise test compartment pressure

Key: Compartment pressure > 30 mmHg

Treatment: Immediate fasciotomy

GOUT

Acute arthritis affecting one joint, which is caused by monosodium urate crystals.

Most commonly seen in obese, middle-aged men but also associated with Lesch-Nyhan syndrome, hyperuricemia, and loop diuretic use.

Presentation: Sudden onset of painful, red, swollen great toe with or without tophi

Diagnostic Test: Joint aspiration reveals *negative birefringent needle–shaped crystals*

Treatment: Acute—colchicine, indomethacin; maintenance—allopurinol, probenecid

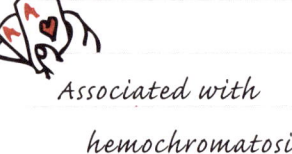

Discontinue any loop diuretic use.

Associated with hemochromatosis

PSEUDOGOUT

Similar to gout except knee is most common joint affected

Diagnostic Test: Joint aspiration reveals *positive birefringent rhomboid crystals*

FIBROMYALGIA

Muscle pain, weakness, fatigue, *without inflammation*

Most common in women over 50 years old

Presentation and Diagnostic Tests: Multiple (> 11–18) tender trigger points

Treatment: NSAIDs, amytryptilline, and cyclobenzaprene

POLYMYOSITIS

Striated muscle inflammation, primarily affects women
Presentation: Symmetric proximal muscle weakness
Key: *Patient will say "difficulty rising from chair"*
Diagnostic Tests: Elevated CK, abnormal EMG
Gold Standard Test: Muscle biopsy
Treatment: High dose steroids

DERMATOMYOSITIS

Polymyositis plus heliotropic rash (red periorbital) and/or
 Grotton's papules (bony prominences on dorsum of
 hand)
Same diagnostic tests and treatment as polymyositis

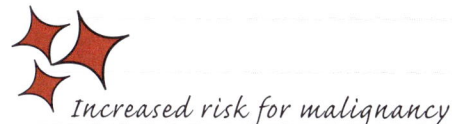

Increased risk for malignancy

PAGET'S DISEASE (OSTEITIS DEFORMANS)

Osteoclasts produce excessive bone turnover.
Presentation: Increased hat size, deafness, leg bowing, with
 or without bone pain or headache
Diagnostic Tests: *X-ray* will show expanded bone cortex
 often referred to as mosaic, marble, or fluffy appearance
Labs: Normal Ca+ and P, increased alk phos and urine
 hydroxyproline
Treatment: Alendronate
Complications: Easy fractures and *secondary osteosarcoma*

X-ray is best, not bone scan,
 because it is a clast problem
 not a blast problem.

TEMPORAL ARTERITIS (GIANT CELL ARTERITIS)

Subacute granulomatous inflammation of large vessels
Presentation: Headache, temporal tenderness, jaw
 claudication
Diagnostic Test: Greatly increased ESR
Gold Standard Test: Temporal artery biopsy
Treatment: If suspect TA, start *high dose steroids* before
 biopsy because a common complication is blindness.
Key: Females over 60 years old; ESR > 60
Treatment: > 60 mg prednisone

POLYMYALGIA RHEUMATICA

Commonly coincides with temporal arteritis and is more common in older women
Presentation: Shoulder and pelvic girdle pain and weakness
Key: Patient complains "can't wave or brush hair"
Diagnostic Tests: Primarily clinical; may see anemia and increased ESR
Treatment: Low-dose prednisone

SCLERODERMA/PROGRESSIVE SYSTEMIC SCLEROSIS

Most common in females 30–50 years old
Presentation: CREST syndrome plus thick skin on face and/or extremities
Diagnostic Tests: Anticentromere Ab—CREST syndrome; antitopoisomerase (Anti Scl-70)—scleroderma
Treatment: Steroids

CREST: Calcinosis, Raynaud's, Esophageal dysmotility, Scleroderma, Telengectasia

SLE

Autoimmune and primarily affects African American women
Presentation: Cytopenias, neurological disturbances, kidney damage, malar/discoid rash, photosensitivity, arthritis, pericarditis, +VDRL or RPR for syphilis
Diagnostic Tests:
> + ANA is not specific.
> +Anti-dsDNA and Anti-Smith are specific.
> +Antihistone AB—drug-induced lupus.
> +Antiphospholipid Ab—recurrent spontaneous abortions.

Treatment: NSAIDs, severe steroids
Complications: Increased risk of spontaneous abortion and congenital complete heart block

OSTEOARTHRITIS

Degenerative joint disease with no systemic manifestations
Primarily affects weight-bearing joints of obese older patients with history of joint trauma
Presentation: Pain in weight-bearing joints, DIPs (Herberden's), and PIPs (Bouchard's)

Worse with activity, better with rest

Diagnostic Tests: Normal labs, x-ray—irregular joint space narrowing with presence of *osteophytes or bone spurs*

Treatment: Weight reduction and NSAIDs

RHEUMATOID ARTHRITIS

Chronic, destructive, inflammatory arthritis plus systemic symptoms (fever, fatigue, subcutaneous nodules)

Most common in women 30–50 years old

Presentation: Symmetric joint involvement with pain, swelling, and stiffness in the morning for more than 1 hour for at least 6 weeks duration

Key: Pannus formation

Diagnostic Tests: Rheumatoid factor positive, synovial fluid 3,000–5,000 WBC/microliter

X-ray: Soft tissue swelling and joint space narrowing

Treatment: NSAIDs, COX-2; if severe, steroids

Most common joints affected:

wrist, MCPs, PIPs

CHAPTER 12 NEUROLOGY

LOBES

- Frontal—motor, UMN lesion, Broca's area, personality, and "home of the hippocampus" (short-term memory)
- Temporal—hearing, balance, hallucinations, Wernicke's area
- Parietal—spacial coordination, cognition
- Occipital—vision

Medulla: Maintains regular heart rate and respiratory rate
Pons: Reacts to environmental changes (respiratory rate, heart rate, apneustic breathing) and is most sensitive to osmotic shifts

HYDROCEPHALUS (TWO TYPES)

Communicating
Excess CSF communicating between ventricles
Newborns—interventricular hemorrhage
Young adult female—pseudotumor cerebri
Elderly—atrophy

Noncommunicating
CSF flow obstruction
Newborn—aqueduct stenosis or Dandy-Walker cyst
Child/young adult—astrocytoma, glioma

PERIPHERAL NEUROPATHIES: SLOWED NERVE CONDUCTION

Trauma: Radial nerve palsy—alcoholic passes out, sleeps on his arm, and puts prolonged pressure on radial nerve
Vitamin B$_1$: (dry beriberi) Wernicke's encephalopathy— ataxia, ophthalmoplegia, encephalopathy
Vitamin B$_{12}$: Seen with pernicious anemia; loss of vibration in lower extremities, positive Babinski, hyperreflexia, ataxia, loss of position sense, spasticity
Vitamin B$_6$: Seen in conjunction with isoniazid treatment; peripheral sensory neuropathy
Vitamin A: Vision loss
Lead: Abdominal and neuro symptoms plus wrist/foot drop
DM: Autonomic and sensory neuropathy

GCS ≥ 14: Minor head injury

GCS from 9–13: Moderate head injury

GCS ≤ 8: Severe head injury

COMA

Causes: Metabolic, medications, endocrine, drug abuse, alcohol abuse, hemorrhage, infarction, abscess, tumor
Treatment: Stabilize—ABCs; treat underlying cause; administer—dextrose, oxygen, naloxone, thiamine

"Locked-In" Syndrome (Persistent Vegetative State)
Awake and alert but can only move eyes and eyelids.
Most common cause—central pontine myelinolysis
Other causes—occlusion of basilar in pons; advanced ALS

Glasgow Coma Scale (Total 15)
Eye opening, motor response, verbal response; see Table 12-1.
(GCS is also featured in Chapter 19, "Surgery.")

TABLE 12-1 Glasgow Coma Scale

Eye Opening		Motor Response		Verbal Response	
Spontaneous	4	Obey	6	Oriented	5
To verbal		Localization	5	Confused	4
commands	3	Flexion	4	Inappropriate	3
To pain	2	Abdominal		Incomprehensible	
None	1	flexion	3	sounds	2
		Extension	2	None	1
		None	1		

DEMENTIA

15% of people older than 65 suffer from dementia.

Alzheimer's Disease
Most common cause of dementia
Most important risk factor—age
Presentation: First amnesia, followed by depression, agitation, aphasia, apraxia
Pathognomonic: Neuritic plaques, neurofibrillary tangles, amyloid deposition
Diagnostic Tests: Clinical; definitive diagnosis can only be made at autopsy
Treatment: Cholinesterase inhibitors
After onset, 5- to 10-year survival

DISEQUILIBRIUM

Equilibrium is maintained by vestibular, visual, cerebellum, brainstem, and proprioception.

S and S: Light-headed, loss of balance, vertigo.

Causes: Ménière's, BBPV, aminoclycosides, furosemide, stroke, acoustic neuroma

See Figure 12-1 for disequilibrium categories.

FIGURE 12-1 Disequilibrium

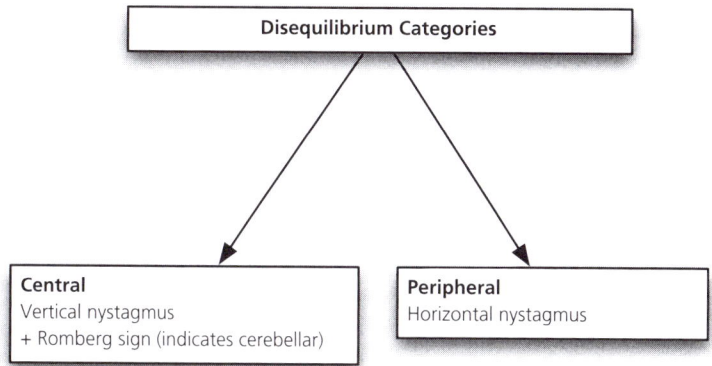

Ménière's Disease

Hearing loss plus vertigo, nausea and vomiting, tinnitus

Resolves in hours–days

Treatment: Antihistamines, acetazolamide

Benign Positional Paroxysmal Vertigo

Nystagmus without hearing loss and vertigo with certain head positions

Episodes last more than 1 minute

Peripheral vertigo

Diagnostic Test: Dix-Hallpike maneuver (turn head to side while going from sitting to supine position)

Resolves weeks–months

Treatment: Supportive

HEADACHES

- New onset headache, focal neurological deficits, or papilledema must be investigated.
- Rule out TA, SAH ("worst headache of my life," LP—grossly bloody CSF), tumor, pseudotumor cerebri (obese girl with HA worse in morning, N/V, –CT papilledema; can cause vision loss).
- Remember HA caused by increased ICP will show papilledema; HA worse in morning, vomiting (possibly projectile).

For suspicion of subarachnoid hemorrhage, see Figure 12-2.

FIGURE 12-2 Suspect Subarachnoid Hemorrhage?

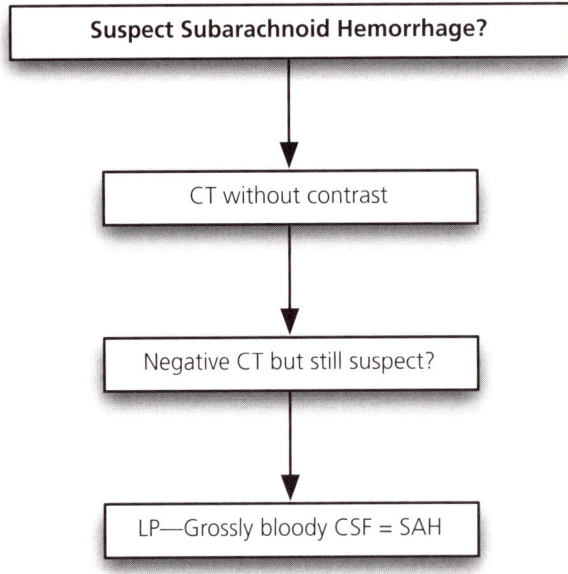

Migraine

More common in women with family history

More than 2 hours of throbbing headache; commonly associated with nausea and vomiting, photophobia, and noise sensitivity

Cause: Unknown etiology

Triggers: Bright light, stress, food, BCPs, menses

Presentation: Pain can be unilateral or bilateral periorbital pain with or without aura, visual changes (commonly light flashes)

Diagnostic Test: Based on history
Suspect something more serious if focal neurological deficits are present (order CT or MRI)
Treatment: Sumatriptan

Cluster

Age of onset: 20–30 years old
More common in men
30 min–3 hours unilateral, periorbital headache
"Cluster" refers to: same time of year, same time of day, same part of head
Exacerbated by alcohol or vasodilating drugs
Presentation: Patient woken up from sleep with unilateral, periorbital headache; ipsilateral tearing, nasal congestion, or Horner's syndrome
Diagnostic Tests: Clinical if classic presentation
Treatment: High-flow O_2

Tension

Most common adult headache
Tight-band-like pain associated with feelings of tightness and stiffness
Diagnostic Test: Diagnosis of exclusion
Treatment: Massage, NSAIDs, avoid triggers

MOVEMENT DISORDERS

Parkinson's Disease

Due to loss of dopamine primarily located in the substantia nigra
Signs and Symptoms:
- Resting "pill-rolling" tremor (stops with sleep or movement)
- Cogwheel rigidity
- Shuffling "festinating" gait
- Masklike facies

Treatment: (first) Bromocriptine; (second) levodopa/carbidopa, selegiline
Surgical Options: Deep brain stimulation, surgical pallidotomy

Idiopathic and hypokinetic
Average age of onset ~ 60 years old

Sudden onset of Parkinsonism in young patient? Suspect MPTP

Huntington's Disease

Autosomal dominant

Abnormal CAG triplet repeat chromosome 4p

Presents 35–50 years old with life expectancy more than 20 years from diagnosis

Presentation: Choreform movements, progressive intellectual deterioration, dementia

Diagnostic Tests: CT/MRI shows *atrophy of caudate nucleus and putamen*

Genetic tests to assess number of CAG repeats (normal < 29)

Treatment: Antipsychotic meds, reserpine for movements, genetic counseling

Seizures

Excessive neuron discharge

Causes: Metabolic disorder, toxins, alcohol, benzo/barbiturate withdrawal, eclampsia, CNS infection, stroke, trauma, congenital, drug OD

More than half of patients experience an aura before seizing.

See Figure 12-3 for determining the cause of seizures.

FIGURE 12-3 Determine Cause of Seizures

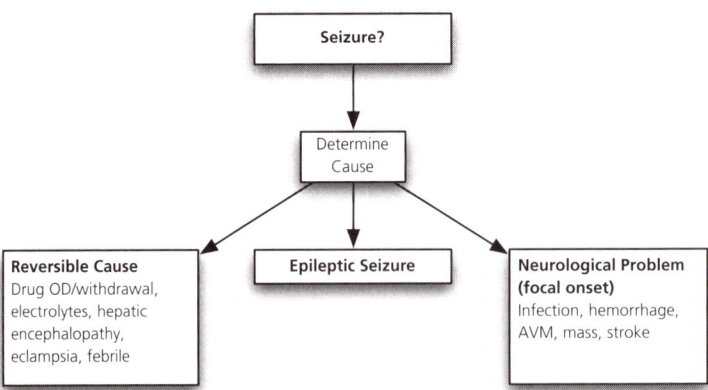

Diagnostic Tests:
1. EEG (considered best test)
2. Rule out systemic causes
3. CT/MRI with contrast

Key: Elevated prolactin = epileptic seizure

The different types of seizures are listed in Table 12-2.

In first-time seizure patients, always rule out reversible causes and masses before starting meds.

Normal EEG does not rule out epilepsy.

TABLE 12-2 Types of Seizures

Partial Seizures					
	Locale	S&S	Key	Postictal	Treatment
Simple partial seizure	Parietal lobe	Manifests as: Psychic (cognitive symptoms) Autonomic (BP, HR) Motor: Jacksonian March Sensory: Hallucinations	No LOC	Possible residual neuro deficit: Todd's palsy (resolves on own)	Kids: Phenobarbitol Adults: Phenytoin, carbamazapine, phenobarbitol, or valproic acid
Complex partial seizure	Temporal lobe	Simple partial plus LOC May mimic acute psychosis: hallucinations, aggressive behavior, tongue writhing	LOC present	Confusion, memory loss	Carbamazepine, phenytoin, or valproate
Generalized Seizures					
	Locale	S&S	Key	Postictal	Treatment
Tonic clonic (grand mal) seizure	Both cerebral hemispheres	First tonic contractions Second clonic contractions, starts in back and limbs Duration: 2–5 minutes	Sudden LOC Incontinence and tongue biting	Muscle ache, headache, confusion	Kids: Phenobarbitol Adults: Valproate
Absence seizure (Always starts before 20 years old)	Both cerebral hemi-spheres	Sudden impaired conciousness around 70 times/ day, with or without associated eye flutter, lip-smacking	Sudden LOC; no loss of muscle tone Classic: Kid in class stops talking midsentence; 20 sec later resumes sentence	Amnesia just before and after	Ethosuximide, valproate

LOC—loss of conciousness. Meds—first-line listed first.
Absence: Patient is usually accused of "daydreaming in school."
Diagnostic for absence: EEG—3 per second spike and wave.

STATUS EPILEPTICUS
Life-threatening medical emergency
Causes: Too rapid withdrawal of anticonvulsants, other drug intoxication, infection, trauma, idiopathic
Diagnostic Criteria:
1. Multiple seizures (any type) follow back-to-back with no return to baseline consciousness
   or
2. Seizure lasting longer than 30 minutes with no periods of consciousness

Diagnostic Tests: Determine underlying cause (toxicology screen, ABG, LFT, Bun/Cr, CBC, electrolytes); wait for patient to stabilize before performing EEG, CT, LP.
Treatment:
1. Stabilize patient (airway, breathing, circulation); prevent aspiration
2. Protect airway, loading-dose phenytoin, IV diazepam (can also try phenobarbitol or sedative)

ADDITIONAL SEIZURES IN CHILDREN

Febrile Seizure
Seizure due to fever in children less than 5 years of age
Presentation: Child with high fever has tonic clonic generalized seizure for less than 3 minutes duration.
Diagnostic Tests: EEG; investigate and rule out other causes of seizure.
Treatment: Treat cause of fever, Children's Tylenol.

Infantile Spasm (West Syndrome)
Onset before 12 months of age
Diagnostic Criteria:
1. Psychomotor development stops at time of syndrome onset
2. Abnormal EEG—slow wave/high amplitude "hypsarrhythmia"
3. Tonic clonic generalized seizures

Seizures occur while tired or just after awakening
Treatment: ACTH, prednisone, and antiepileptics

TREMOR/CHOREA

See Table 12-3 for information about types of tremor/chorea.

Febrile seizure is not a diagnosis of epilepsy!

Infantile Spasm—Key Terms
Baby < 1 year old with seizure:
- *Occurs when drowsy*
- *EEG—hypsarrhythmia*
- *Treat—ACTH*

All anticonvulsants are teratogenic.
Child-bearing age? Pregnancy test before prescribing.
Advise patients not to become pregnant.

TABLE 12-3 Tremor/Chorea

Type of Tremor/Chorea	Area
Resting tremor Stops with rest or initiation of sleep **Causes:** Drug intoxication or withdrawal, anxiety Parkinson's disease—pill-rolling resting tremor Benign essential hereditary tremor—AD, plus family history (treat with B-blockers)	**Basal ganglia disease**
Intention Tremor	**Cerebellar disease**
Asterixis Outstretched hand-flapping	**Kidney or liver disease**
Hemiballismus Hemi- means half; half your body's limbs flail uncontrollably	**Subthalamic nucleus lesion**

WEAKNESS

Carpal Tunnel Syndrome
Median nerve compression
Average age: Around 40 years old
More common in women
Cause: Repetitive use injury (typing, etc.)
Presentation: Affects thumb, index, middle, lateral half ring finger—numbness, tingling, weakness alleviated by shaking out hands
Diagnostic Tests:
      Tinel's sign—tingling sensation upon tapping wrist over median nerve
      Phalen's sign—pain with 90-degree wrist flexion for 30 seconds
      Confirmatory—EMG, nerve conduction velocity
Treatment: Wrist splints, NSAIDs, alleviate repetitive cause; surgery—carpal tunnel release

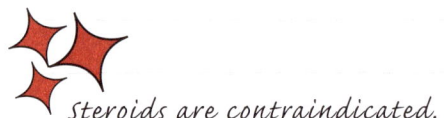

Steroids are contraindicated.

Guillain-Barré Syndrome

Mild infection 12 weeks ago (*Campylobacter jejuni*)

Presentation:
>Distal symmetric weakness/paralysis
>Loss of DTRs
>Ascending paralysis
>Watch closely—may have to ventilate

Diagnostic Tests: CSF—protein < 55 mg/dL with *no* pleocytosis

Treatment: Mild—usually resolves on own with complete recovery; severe—plasmapheresis shortens illness time

Myasthenia Gravis

Autoimmune; more common in young women

Antiacetylcholine Ab's vs postsynaptic Ach receptors

Presentation: Muscle fatigue, ptosis, diplopia (ocular muscle weakness)

Key: "Symptoms get worse through the day"; associated with *thymoma* and other autoimmune disorders

Diagnostic Tests: "Tensilon" edrophonium administration—improves symptom (short acting); decreased response to repetitive nerve stimulus

Treatment:
>Neostigmine, pyridostigmine, steroids
>Severe—IVIG, plasmapheresis
>*Curative*—thymoma resection

Myasthetic-Like Syndrome

Excess parasympathetics (diarrhea, urinary urgency, miosis, bronchial secretions) plus muscle weakness (like in myasthenia)

Cause: Organophosphate poisoning

Edrophonium exacerbates muscle weakness

Treatment: Pralidoxime and atropine

Eaton-Lambert Syndrome

Caused by impaired Ach release

Presentation: Paraneoplastic seen with lung small cell CA, muscle weakness but spares ocular muscles

Improves with muscle stimulation

Amyotrophic Lateral Sclerosis

See Table 12-4.

Idiopathic, progressive, neurodegenerative

Age of onset: Around 55 years old

More common in males

Diagnostic Criteria: Upper and lower motor neuron lesions in three or more organs

UMN—positive Babinski's, hyperreflexia, spasticity

LMN—atrophy, flaccidity, fasciculations

EMG—fib potentials, widespread denervation

Treatment: Supportive; after onset, only a few years until death

Multiple Sclerosis

See Table 12-4.

Progressive T-mediated autoimmune demyelinating disease

Peak age of onset: 20–40 years old

Predominantly female

Presentation:

"Waxing and waning" symptoms

Vertigo, limb weakness, scanning speech, gait disturbance, incontinence, mental status changes

Eye: Diplopia, internuclear ophthalmoplegia, nystagmus

Diagnostic Tests: MRI—gadolinium shows demyelinating plaques; CSF—increased IgG, myelin basic proteins, oligoclonal bands; corpus callosum lesions

Treatment: Steroids, interferons

MULTIPLE SCLEROSIS KEYS TO DIAGNOSIS

20–40-year-old woman with ocular, mental status, or neurologic changes

MRI—demyelinating plaques

CSF—IgG, mbp's, oligoclonal bands

Corpus callosum lesions

TABLE 12-4 Lesions of the Spinal Cord

Syringomyelia	May be caused by cranial malformations or trauma—cervical or thoracic central cavitation of spinal cord
	Presentation: "Cape distribution" loss of pain and temperature sense below lesion
	Diagnostic Test: MRI
	Treatment: Shunt via surgery
Brown-Séquard syndrome (hemisection)	Clean cut injury
	Contralateral loss of pain sensation distal to injury, ipsilateral paralysis and loss of proprioception
Multiple sclerosis	Random asymmetric lesions
ALS	No sensory deficit
	LMN plus UMN deficits present
Werdnig Hoffmann	Spares ocular muscles
	Flaccid paralysis plus LMN lesion

BRAIN LESIONS

For lesions of the brain, see Table 12-5 and Table 12-6.

TABLE 12-5 Localizing Lesions of the Brain

Localizing Lesions Deficit	Area
Broca's aphasia	Frontal lobe
Wernicke's aphasia	Temporal lobe
No read, write, or arithmetic	Parietal lobe
Ignore contralateral half of body and world	Parietal lobe
Visual hallucinations	Occipital lobe
Personality changes	Frontal lobe
Kluver-Bucy syndrome—hyperorality and hypersexuality	Bilateral amygdala
Wernicke-Korsakoff's syndrome—alcoholic anterograde amnesia plus confabulations	Bilateral mamillary bodies
Ataxia, nystagmus, scanning speech, intention tremor	Cerebellum

TABLE 12-6 Upper Motor Neuron vs. Lower Motor Neuron Lesions

LMN Lesion	Decreased DTRs	Atrophy	Flaccid paralysis	Fasciculations
UMN Lesion	Hyperactive DTRs	Minor atrophy	Spastic paralysis	+ Babinski

"TJ Hooker"—ipsilateral deviations

CN12—ipsilateral Tongue deviation

CN5—ipsilateral Jaw deviation

CN 11—ipsilateral Head deviation

CN 3, 4—Midbrain; CN 5, 6, 7, 8—Pons; CN 9, 10, 11, 12—Medulla

CN 1—Kallman's syndrome: hypogonadism plus anosmia

CN 5—Trigeminal neuralgia: ipsilateral shooting facial pain; treat: amitriptyline

CN 7—Bell's palsy: UMN—ipsilateral forehead spared

CN 8—Deafness, tinnitus

CN 9—Taste loss (posterior third of tongue) plus loss of gag

CN 5—Hoarse, dysphagia, loss of gag

CN 10—Contralateral uvula deviation

Unilateral cerebellum—ipsilateral fall

APHASIAS

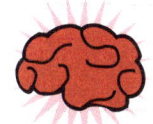

Broca's
(Expressive) motor aphasia; comprehension intact

Wernicke's
(Receptive) sensory aphasia; poor comprehension and speaks nonsense

Expressive because patient cannot express themselves. Receptive because patient cannot receive language.

TRANSIENT ISCHEMIC ATTACK (TIA)

Commonly a precursor for impending stroke

Causes: Short-term neurological deficit (minutes–hours) that resolves spontaneously; commonly due to carotid stenosis

Presentation: Amaurosis fugax (occlusion of ophthalmic artery = ipsilateral blindness), and/or unilateral weakness; carotid bruit heard

Diagnostic Test: U/S or duplex scan of carotid artery

Treatment:

    Stenosis < 70% = daily aspirin

    Stenosis > 70% = carotid endarterectomy if patient is stable (best long-term prognosis)

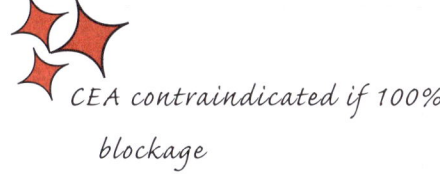

CEA contraindicated if 100% blockage

STROKE

Neurologic deficit due to low blood flow

Two Types:

- Ischemic stroke (vast majority)
- Hemorrhagic stroke (less common)

Risk Factors: DM, hypercholesterolemia, hypercoaguability, HTN, obesity, smoking, IVDU, atrial fibrillation

Lateral striate are commonly affected.

Causes:

- Atherosclerosis (associated with carotid stenosis)
- Lacunar infarcts (small vessels)
- Any condition that predisposes to emboli formation
- IVDU-endocarditis-septic emboli
- Atrial fibrillation (very common)
- Congenital cardiac anomalies
- Valvular disease

Diagnostic Tests:

1. CT *without* contrast—hemorrhagic stroke (bright white) vs ischemic stroke (black)
2. MRI—reveals extent of damage from early ischemic stroke

Other Studies:
- ECG and ECHO if suspect embolic stroke
- Transesophageal echo (TEE)—mural thrombi
- Follow TIA investigation in the preceding section—extracranial disease
- Magnetic resonance angio (MRA)—intracranial disease

Initial Treatment:
Allow BP to rise to maintain cerebral perfusion pressure.
ASA if onset in > 48 hours (do not administer if currently on tPA).
tPA: Onset of symptoms within 3 hours of *ischemic* stroke (contraindicated with hemorrhagic stroke).

Many Contraindications to tPA Use:
- Age < 18 years old
- Seizure at onset of stroke symptoms
- Any recent history of bleeding or predisposition to bleeding
- Low platelets, surgery in past 2 weeks, etc.
- Systolic BP > 185
- Diastolic BP >110

Long-Term Treatment:
Treat modifiable risk factors: HTN, DM, etc.
CEA if applicable (best long-term survival rate); *see previous TIA section*
Anticoagulation if hemorrhagic type is absolutely ruled out!
ASA—especially if stroke due to small vessel disease

VON HIPPEL-LINDAU DISEASE

VHL drives a "CAR"

Cerebellar hemangioblastoma

AD (family history)

Retinal angiomas

AD—family history
Presentation: Headache, N and V
Neoplasms/Possible Manifestations:
1. Renal cell CA—polycythemia due to increase in erythropoietin
2. Pheochromocytoma—catecholamines
3. Cerebellar hemangioblastoma—cerebellar signs
4. Retinal angioma

Diagnostic Tests: CT—posterior fossa mass with or without densities
Treatment: Surgery

OSLER-WEBER-RENDU SYNDROME

AD—family history

Telengectasias, AVMs, and aneurysms: Lung, GI, brain

Presentation: Brain—cerebral embolism or abscess; lung—hypoxemia; GI—abdominal pulsatile mass, painless bleeding

Treatment: Supportive treatment

INCREASED INTRACRANIAL PRESSURE (ICP)

HA, N and V, papilledema, bilateral fixed and dilated pupils

Treatment: Intubate, hyperventilate, and reverse Trendelenberg

NEUROLOGY BLEEDS

For additional information on neurology bleeds, refer to Chapter 19, "Surgery."

Epidural Hematoma

Usually caused by blow to side of head involving temporal bone causing bleeding from middle meningeal artery.

Biconvex shaped

Presentation: Head trauma followed by *"lucid interval"* and then loss of consciousness

>   Around half of these patients present with ipsilateral blown pupil, which is a sign of increased ICP; therefore spinal tap is contraindicated because it may cause uncal herniation.

Diagnostic Test: CT without contrast

Treatment: Craniotomy and decompression

Subdural Hematoma

Caused by head trauma that leads to bleeding of bridging veins in cortex and dural sinus.

Crescent shaped

Presentation: Classic scenario is *"alcoholic who bumps head"* and presents 1–2 weeks later with neurologic deterioration. Patient may present up to 2 months after insult.

Diagnostic Test: CT without contrast

Treatment: Surgical evacuation

Any signs of increased ICP = contraindication spinal tap, get CT first

Suspect neurological bleed? Always order CT without contrast; blood—bright white

Subarachnoid Hemorrhage
Caused by trauma or ruptured berry aneurysm causing
blood flow between arachnoid and pia mater.
Presentation: *"Worst headache of my life"* is the key
phrase; patient may also have positive Kernig's and
Brudzinski's signs
Diagnostic Test: First CT without contrast (best choice);
(only if CT is inconclusive) LP—reveals grossly bloody CSF
(not highly recommended)
Cerebral angiogram can locate the defect for surgical
intervention.
Treatment: Anticonvulsants, nimodipine

Intracerebral Hemorrhage
Common causes are hypertension and a/v malformations,
which cause bleeding in parenchyma.
Bleeding in basal ganglia is commonly associated with HTN.
Causes: HTN, AVM, tumor
Presentation: Contralateral hemisensory deficits and
hemiplegia
Diagnostic Test: CT without contrast
Treatment: If possible, surgery

Cushing's Reflex
Treatment: Make changes in MAP or ICP to keep CPP
constant; give mannitol, acetazolamide (decreases MAP);
ventilate with O_2 (decreases PO_2 and ICP)

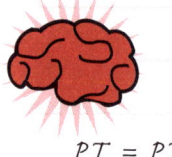

Must keep CPP constant!

Mean Arterial Pressure

– IntraCranial Pressure =

Cerebral Perfusion Pressure

MAP – ICP = CPP

PT = PT

TRACTS

- Corticospinal—begins in cortex, UMN lesions
- Spinocerebellar—gait, depth perception, intention
  tremor, vertical nystagmus, left dysmetria (no finger
  to nose or heel to shin)
- Subthalamic—fine motor coordination, left
  hemiballismus
- SpinoThalamic—Pain and Temperature, crosses in the
  cord

NEUROFIBROMATOSIS

Both types will have family history

Type 1
Chromosome 17 (Von Recklinhausen's)

Need two or more of the following positive for diagnosis:

1. Optic glioma
2. Freckling
3. Six café au lait spots (> 15 mm adults, > 5 mm kids)
4. Two Lisch nodules (pigmented iris hamartoma)

Type 2
Chromosome 22
Bilateral acoustic neuroma

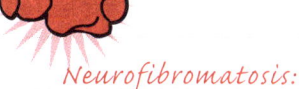

Neurofibromatosis:

Type 1: Cx 17 (Von
  Recklinhausen's)

17 letters

Type 2: Cx 22

2 acoustic neuromas

TUBEROUS SCLEROSIS

Mental retardation and infantile spasms *plus* ash-leaf hypopigmented lesions; sebaceous adenoma; small, red nodules on cheeks, nose

Diagnostic Tests: CT—calcified tubers in periventricular areas

NEUROLOGICAL NEOPLASMS

See Table 12-7.

TABLE 12-7 Neurological Neoplasms

Tumor	S&S	Treatment
GBM (grade IV astrocytoma)	MC primary brain tumor —Increased ICP symptoms Rapid course/poor prognosis	Surgery, radiation, chemo
Meningioma	Arachnoid or dura —Good prognosis	Radiation, surgery
Acoustic neuroma	Schwann cells —Same-side hearing loss	Surgery
Childhood onset		
Astrocytoma	Increased ICP symptoms with or without same-side paralysis —Prognosis better than GBM	Surgery, radiation
Medulloblastoma	Fourth ventricle —Increased ICP symptoms —Super malignant	Chemo, radiation, surgery
Ependymoma	Fourth ventricle or spinal cord —Hydrocephalus	Radiation, surgery

CHAPTER 13 OBSTETRICS

HCG

Used to detect pregnancy; positive after 8 days.
Acts like LH and maintains corpus luteum during first trimester.
With abnormally elevated HCG always consider hydatiform mole.
See Figure 13-1 for a description of implantation.

FIGURE 13-1 Implantation

Cytotrophoblast	+	Trophoblast	=	Synctiotrophoblast
(Mom's wall)		(Baby)		(Mom, baby, and chorion)

PREGNANCY DATING

280 days since conception
42 weeks since last menstrual period

Nagele's rule: LMP + 9 months + 7 days = due date

NORMAL FETAL HEART RATE

120–160 bpm

WAYS TO DETERMINE GESTATIONAL AGE

1. Uterine size
2. Quickening—first fetal movements detected by mother
3. Fetal heart tones (10 weeks via Doppler)
4. U/S 5–12 weeks crown/rump length or biparietal diameter 16–20 weeks (most accurate)

Normal weight gain of pregnancy: around 30 lb

DIETARY SUPPLEMENTS

1 mg folate daily
30–60 mg iron daily

Calcium deficiency presents as leg cramps in pregnant females.

SURGERY IN PREGNANCY

Elective Surgery: Avoid until after delivery.
Semi-Urgent Condition: Wait until second trimester.
Urgent Life-Threatening Condition: Operate; proceed in the same manner as you would with patients who are not pregnant.

Pregnancy Dates:
>   38 weeks = term
>   More than 42 weeks = post-term
>   20–37 weeks = preterm
>   36 weeks = lung maturity
>   Abortion = termination at less than 20 weeks gestation
>   or fetal weight less than 500 gm

See Table 13-1 for teratogens and their possible effects.

TABLE 13-1 Teratogens

Drug	Effects
DES	Cervical incompetence, clear cell adenocarcinoma
Diazepam	Cleft lip/palate
Tetracycline	Gray/brown tooth discoloration
Aminoglycosides	Deafness
Valproic acid	Neural tube defects
Cigarettes	Low birth weight, prematurity
Cocaine	Mental retardation
Warfarin	IUGR, stillbirths
BCPs	VACTERL
Phenytoin	Microcephaly, mental retardation
Isotretinoin	Craniofacial, CVS, CNS malformations
Lithium	Epstein's anomaly
ACE	Oligohydramnios
Methotrexate	IUGR

Fetal Alcohol Syndrome: Microcephaly, limb dislocations, facial abnormalities, heart and lung abnormalities
Highest Risk: 3–8 weeks after conception
>   Most common cause of preventable congenital malformation

NORMAL PHYSIOLOGIC CHANGES IN PREGNANCY

Hematologic: Decreased hemoglobin and hematocrit, increased plasma volume
>   The increased plasma volume causes a physiologic anemia.
>   However, hemoglobin less than 11 is not normal.

CV: Blood pressure decreases (both systolic and diastolic components)

Increased cardiac output, heart rate, and stroke volume

Chest x-ray = cardiomegaly

Respiratory: *Respiratory rate is unchanged.*

Increased tidal volume and minute ventilation.

Increased pO_2 and decreased pCO_2

Renal: Increased GFR and increased aldosterone

Skin/Vagina: Striae, linea nigra present, vagina shows Chadwick's sign (violet color)

SIZE/DATE DISCREPANCY

At 20–35 weeks number of cm's should = number of weeks

2-to-3–cm difference = size/date discrepancy

Evaluation: U/S

Three Compartments of Uterus:

1. Fetal dimensions: biparietal diameter, head circumference, abdominal circumference, femur length
2. Amniotic fluid: 5–25 amniotic fluid index is normal range
3. Placenta
   - When assessing size/date discrepancy, the most useful tool is U/S.
   - Fetal dimensions are important for differentiating between symmetric and asymmetric discrepancies.
   - Amniotic fluid is assessed in all four quadrants.

SGA

SGA is defined as below 10th percentile for fetal age (see Figure 13-2). There are three main types or causes of SGA: fetal (symmetric and asymmetric IUGR), amniotic (oligohydramnios and PROM), and placental.

FIGURE 13-2 Small for Gestational Age (Fetal, Amniotic Fluid, or Placental in Origin) < 10th Percentile for Age

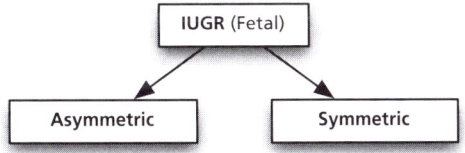

SYMMETRIC IUGR

All four bimetric measurements (fetal dimensions) are decreased.

Cause: Fetal in origin (aneuploidy, trisomy, fetal infection, ToRCHeS); decreased growth potential

Onset: Early in pregnancy

ASYMMETRIC IUGR

Only abdominal circumference is decreased (fetal weight primarily affected by abdomen).

Most common type of IUGR because it is "brain sparing."

Cause: Placental problem (risks are smoking mother, hypertension, and decreased nutrition)

Onset: Late in pregnancy (growth curve is normal until around 30 weeks)

OLIGOHYDRAMNIOS

U/S reveals amniotic fluid index < 5

Indication for delivery

Cause: Fetal urinary tract anomaly or obstruction (fetus cannot add to amniotic fluid causing decreased amount)

PREMATURE RUPTURE OF MEMBRANES (PROM)

Diagnosed by speculum; reveals pooling of fluid, positive nitrazine test (indicated by blue nitrazine paper) and "ferning pattern" of fluid on glass slide

Medications that decrease amniotic fluid: indomethacin and ACE inhibitors

PLACENTAL INSUFFICIENCY

Causes decreased blood flow to fetus, which causes decreased urine production (i.e., decreased amount of amniotic fluid and asymmetric IUGR)

LGA

There are three main causes or origins of LGA:

Fetal—gestational DM, macrosomia, multiple gestation

Amniotic fluid—"polyhydramnios" and its causes

Placental—moles, leiomyomas

Figure 13-3 shows the possible causes for LGA.

FIGURE 13-3 Large for Gestational Age

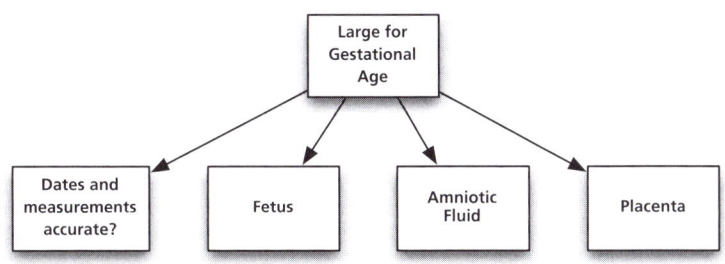

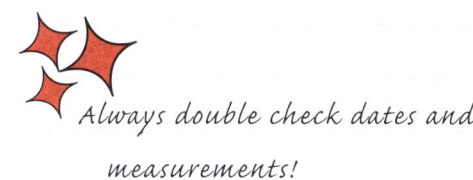

Always double check dates and measurements!

FETUS
Multiple gestation: More babies need more room.
Macrosomia: (Big baby) due to prolonged pregnancy (symmetric)
Gestational Diabetes: Causes large abdomen (asymmetric)

POLYHYDRAMNIOS
Amniotic Fluid: AFI > 25
Cause: Any fetal GI tract anomaly (atresias or fistulas) that prevents baby from swallowing, which causes increased amniotic fluid

DUODENAL ATRESIA
Common in Down's syndrome

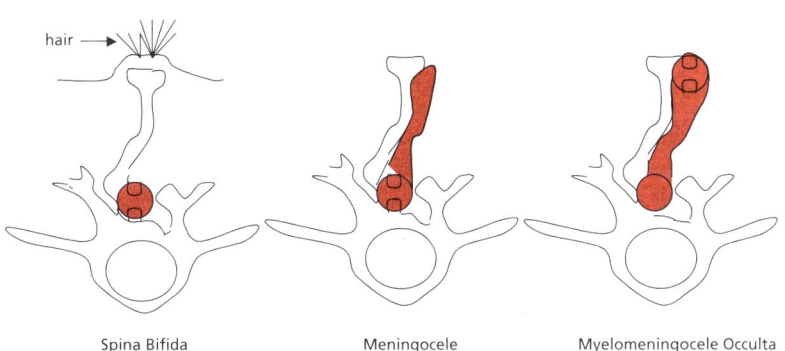

U/S shows "double bubble" sign

NEURAL TUBE DEFECTS
Fetal CSF leaks causing increase in amniotic fluid.
Spina bifida, encephaly (preventable by folate supplementation); see Figure 13-4.

FIGURE 13-4 Common Neural Tube Defects Associated with Polyhydramnios

Spina Bifida Meningocele Myelomeningocele Occulta

Leiomyomas are three times more common in African American women.

Fetal mortality increases by 3% in prolonged pregnancy.

Treatment of post-dates:

If cervix is favorable = induce labor

If cervix is unfavorable = perform NST (nonstress test) and BPP (biophysical profile) twice daily

FETAL HYDROPS
Immune cause: Abnormal antibodies
Key words: Anti D, cal, duffy
Nonimmune Cause: Infection (syphilis)

Placental
Mole: Hypertension early in pregnancy, greatly increased HCG, snowstorm pattern on x-ray
Leiomyoma: Increased estrogen during pregnancy makes leiomyomas grow very large.

POST-DATES COMPLICATIONS

Greater than 42 weeks gestation:
First assess whether or not dates are accurate.
Commonly associated with placental sulfatase deficiency and anencephaly.
If placenta function is maintained in post-dates, it commonly leads to macrosomia and difficult delivery due to large fetus.
If placenta function decreases, **dysmaturity syndrome** can occur:

Acidosis, decreased baby fat, increased risk of meconium aspiration

BLEEDING DURING PREGNANCY

For first trimester bleeding and pregnancy loss, see Figure 13-5.

FIGURE 13-5 First Trimester Bleeding/Loss

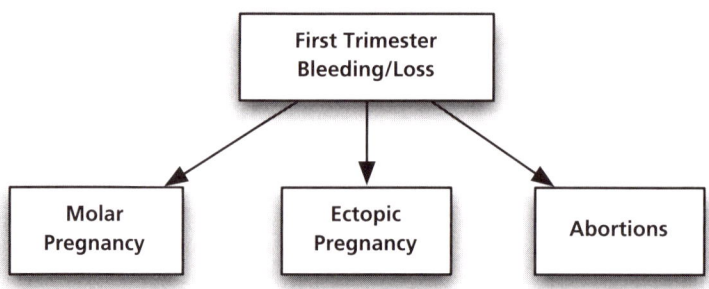

Ectopic Pregnancy
Abdominal pain plus light vaginal bleeding (see Chapter 8, "Gynecology")
Diagnostic Test: U/S to visualize or laparoscopy

Hydatiform Mole
Commonly presents with very elevated HCG, large uterus, and hypertension early in pregnancy
Diagnostic Test: U/S = snowstorm pattern
Treatment: Suction curettage, put patient on BCPs, and follow HCG levels

Abortions
See Chapter 8, Table 8-1.

For second trimester bleeding and pregnancy loss, see Figure 13-6.

FIGURE 13-6 Second Trimester Bleeding and Pregnancy Loss

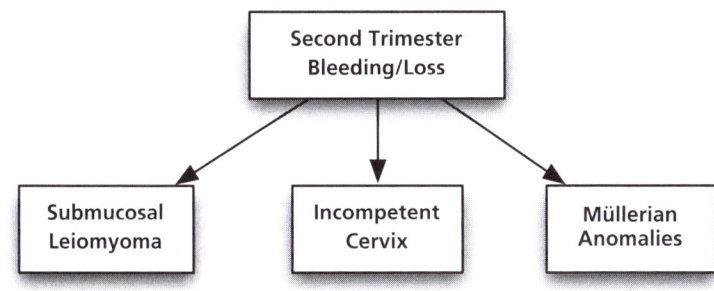

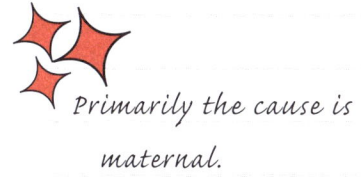
Primarily the cause is maternal.

Submucosal Leiomyoma
Nonviable gestational age
Placenta implants on leiomyoma, which decreases blood flow to fetus
Diagnostic Test: Hysteroscopy or hysterosalpingogram shows deformed uterine cavity
Treatment: Hysteroscopic resection

Delivery of stillborn normal fetus

Incompetent Cervix
Nonviable gestational age (> 24 weeks)
Presentation: Pain*less* cervical dilation and no contractions
Treatment: Subsequent pregnancies require cervical cerclage at 14 weeks

Delivery of immature, normal fetus

Regular painful contractions, cervical dilation, delivery of immature fetus that does not survive

Pay attention to status of painful vs not painful bleeding

Müllerian Anomaly
History of septate or double uterus
Diagnostic Test: Hysteroscopy or hysterosalpingogram
Treatment: Surgery to correct deformity

For third trimester bleeding and pregnancy loss, see Figure 13-7.

FIGURE 13-7 Third Trimester Bleeding

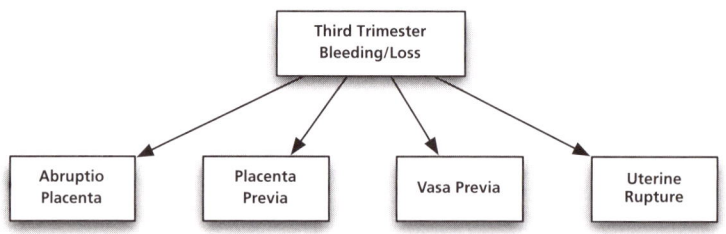

Abruptio Placenta
Pain*ful* dark red bleeding
Risks: Cocaine use, hypertension, trauma
Associated with DIC
Diagnostic Test: U/S only 50% sensitive; primarily *clinical* diagnosis
Treatment:
> Mom and fetus stable at 30 weeks = Conservative
> Mom and fetus unstable = Vaginal delivery
> Mom and fetus in demise = C-section

Placenta Previa
Pain*less* bright red vaginal bleeding
Abnormal placental implantation
Risks: Previous previa, previous or current twin pregnancy, multiparity, maternal age > 35 years
Diagnostic Test: *U/S = placenta in lower segment, no vaginal exam*
Treatment:
> Mom and fetus stable = Scheduled C-section
> Mom and fetus unstable = Emergency C-section

Vasa Previa
Pain*less* vaginal bleeding (fetal in origin)
Risk Factors: Multiple gestation (*the higher the number of fetuses = the higher the risk*) and presence of accessory placenta lobe
Treatment: Immediate C-section; **very life-threatening for fetus**

Vasa previa diagnosis triad:
Artificial rupture of
  membranes
Vaginal bleeding
Fetal bradycardia
"Antepartum hemorrhage with
  fetal bradycardia"

Uterine Rupture

Pain*ful* vaginal bleeding plus uterine contractions and unstable fetal heart pattern

Risks: Previous classic C-section, too much oxytocin administered too quickly, trauma

Complete uterine rupture: Fetus is in abdominal cavity

Incomplete uterine rupture: Peritoneal covering, fetus still in uterus

Diagnostic Test: Fetal parts felt in abdomen

Treatment: Immediate C-section

HYPERTENSION IN PREGNANCY

Mg Sulfate

Prevents seizures and is safe for pregnant women (drug of choice for tocolysis)

Antidote: IV calcium gluconate

Warning! Watch for magnesium toxicity (decreased respiratory rate, decreased DTRs, and possible coma).

Preeclampsia

New onset hypertension (BP over 140/90), at more than 20 weeks gestation

Associated Symptoms: Edema and proteinuria

Treatment: Try to keep diastolic 90–100
>   If preterm, treat with bed rest and observation
>   If near term, check fetal lung maturity; if mature, treat with labor induction

Severe Preeclampsia

Same presentation as mild preeclampsia plus RUQ pain, headache, increased DTRs, and visual changes

Treatment: Hydralazine, steroids, Mg sulfate
>   If preterm (before 36 weeks), conservative treatment with close observation (inpatient)
>   If after 36 weeks, deliver

HELLPs

RUQ pain and increased AST due to hemolysis

Treatment: Hydralazine, steroids, Mg sulfate

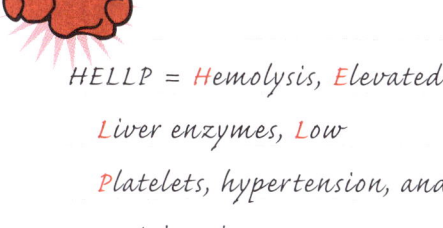

HELLP = Hemolysis, Elevated Liver enzymes, Low Platelets, hypertension, and proteinuria

Chronic Hypertension

Onset of high BP before 20 weeks gestation or prepartum

Treatment: Methyldopa

UTIS IN PREGNANCY

Asymptomatic Bacteriuria
Screen at every checkup in pregnant women
Diagnostic Test: U/A > 100,000 CFU
Treatment: Nitrofurantoin (outpatient)

Acute Cystitis
Dysuria, increased frequency and urgency
Diagnostic Test: Positive culture
Treatment: Antibiotics (outpatient)

Acute Pyelonephritis
Treat aggressively in pregnant women
Presentation: Dysuria, increased frequency and urgency
plus chills and fever, flank pain, *CVA tenderness*
Treatment: Inpatient, IV fluid, cephalosporin; follow-up IVP
after delivery

OTHER PROBLEMS DURING PREGNANCY

Diabetes Mellitus
Preexisting Type I or Type II diabetes before becoming
pregnant
Type I and II: Fetal anomalies (increased risk of cardiac
defects, neural tube defects, and sacral agenesis)
Treatment: Check blood sugar and insulin (oral
hypoglycemics are contraindicated in pregnancy)

Gestational Diabetes Mellitus
Onset at more than 20 weeks gestation; caused by
placental action.
Not associated with fetal anomalies.
Test for GDM at 24–28 weeks.
Fasting Blood Glucose: > 126 or suspect with random blood
glucose > 200
Screen: 1 hour 50g GTT > 140
Confirm: 3 hour 100g GTT with any 2 of the following:
    Fasting > 95
    1 hour > 180
    2 hour > 155
    3 hour > 140

Pregnant Patients with Toxoplasmosis
Treatment:
> First trimester = elective termination or spiramycin
> Second or third trimester = pyramethamine and
> sulfadiazine

Anemia of Pregnancy
Physiologic anemia due to greatly increased plasma volume
is normal during pregnancy; therefore, in order to
diagnose iron deficiency anemia in a pregnant patient
her Hb must be less than or equal to 10 mg/dL.
Iron deficiency anemia has no detrimental effect on fetus.
Folate deficiency causes low birth weight and neural tube
defects.

Sickle Cell Anemia
Carries increased risk of spontaneous abortion, IUGR, and
stillbirth
Diagnostic Test: Hemoglobin electrophoresis (Hb S > 40%
SCA; Hb S < 40% SCA trait)

SLE
Increased risk of spontaneous abortion
Antiphospholipid antibodies
Treatment: Low-dose aspirin in subsequent pregnancies

Morning Sickness
Nausea and vomiting in first trimester

Hyperemesis Gravidum
Severe nausea and vomiting beyond 14–16 weeks gestation
resulting in poor weight gain and dehydration
Cause: Highly elevated HCG; commonly seen with moles
Treatment: IV fluids, frequent small meals

Cholestasis
Jaundice, itching, increased LFTs during pregnancy
Treatment: Cholysteramine
Cure: Delivery

Fatty Liver
Very dangerous condition; onset in third trimester or
postpartum
Treatment: Glucose, fluids, and fresh frozen plasma

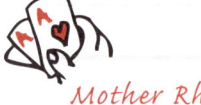

Mother Rh–

Fetus Rh+?

Give RhoGAM at 28 wks and
within 72 hrs after delivery
or any procedure with
chance of transplacental
hemorrhage.

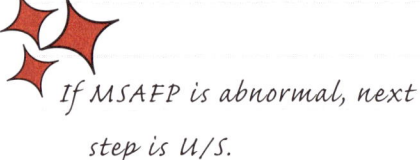

Pregnancy has protective effect
against multiple sclerosis
and peptic ulcer disease.

If MSAFP is abnormal, next
step is U/S.

Rh Incompatibility

Mother Rh+/Fetus Rh–

If mother and father are Rh–, there is no risk.

If father is Rh+ or status unknown, the infant has 50/50 chance of Rh+.

Month 7–delivery: Check Rh antibody titers.

Previous sensitization is required for disease (previous pregnancy).

ANOMALY DETECTION

10–12 Weeks Chorionic Villus Sampling

Only detects chromosomal abnormalities; does not detect neural tube defects.

Good because detects abnormalities early.

Carries a risk of limb defects.

15–20 Weeks Triple Screen or AFP

Detects all neural tube defects and chromosomal abnormalities.

Triple screen (AFP, estriol, HCG) has higher sensitivity vs AFP alone.

Trisomy 21: AFP and estriol are decreased and HCG is increased.

15–17 Weeks Amniocentesis

Detects chromosomal abnormalities and neural tube defects.

Risk of amniotic fluid embolism.

Detects fetal lung maturity.

Routinely used in women older than 35.

Second or Third Trimester PUBS

Collects blood from umbilical cord vessels.

This test can determine fetal karyotype and detect presence of infection.

It is useful in the evaluation and treatment of Rh disease.

STAGES OF NORMAL LABOR

Never admit until patient is at least 3 cm dilated.

Bloody Show: Blood-tinged mucous plug marks onset of labor—*normal occurrence*

Stage 1

LATENT PHASE
Onset of regular contractions
Cervical dilation < 3 cm
Duration: 20 hours primipara; 14 hours multipara

ACTIVE PHASE
Cervical dilation > 3–4 cm
Rate of Dilation: 1.2 cm/hr in primipara patients; 1.5 cm/hr in multipara patients

Stage 2
Complete cervical dilation → delivery of fetus
Duration: 30 minutes–3 hours in primipara patients; 5 minutes–30 minutes in multipara patients

Stage 3
Delivery of infant to delivery of placenta
Rate of delivery: 30 minutes

ABNORMAL LABOR

Prolonged Latent Phase
Cervical dilation < 3 cm
More than 20 hours in primipara patients
More than 14 hours in multipara patients
Cause: Most commonly caused by injudicious anesthesia
Treatment: *Not* C-section

Prolonged or Arrested Active Phase
Cervical dilation > 3 cm

PROLONGED ACTIVE PHASE
Cervical dilation < 1.2 cm/hr primipara; < 1.5 cm/hr multipara
Cause: Cephalopelvic disproportion
Treatment: Oxytocin

ACTIVE PHASE ARREST
No change in more than 2 hours
Treatment: Oxytocin; if no progress in more than 2 hours, C-section

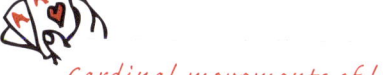

Cardinal movements of labor:

Descent

Flexion

Internal rotation

External rotation

Extension

Expulsion

Lack of FHR acceleration seen in the following: fetal sleeping, CNS anomaly, maternal sedative or narcotic administration, gestational age < 30 weeks

BPP 8–10: normal

BPP below 6: CST

BPP below 4: C-section

Rule of 60s: (severe) HR decreases below 60 and does not increase for 60 seconds

ARREST OF DESCENT

Cervical dilation of 10 cm and 2 hours pass with no delivery

Cause: Midpelvic contractions indicated by "prominent ischial spines"

Treatment: Vacuum, forceps, or C-section

TESTS OF FETAL WELL-BEING (NST, BPP, CST)

Non Stress Test

Fetal heart rate > 15 bpm over baseline for 15 seconds

At least 2 accelerations in 20-minute period

Biophysical Profile

For each parameter, score of 2 is normal and score of 0 is abnormal

    Fetal Tone

    Fetal Breathing (30 breaths in 10 minutes)

    Fetal Movement (3 movements in 10 minutes)

    Amniotic Fluid Index (5–25 is normal)

    Non Stress Test

Contraction Stress Test

Assesses uteroplacental dysfunction

FHR is monitored during contractions

Repetitive late deceleration (3 in 10 minutes) = concern about fetus

Early Deceleration

Simultaneous deceleration with contraction

Cause: Head compression (normal, no distress)

Variable Deceleration

No predictability of FHR with onset of contraction

Cause: Umbilical cord compression (change mother's position)

HR drops below 60 bpm

HR drops 60 beats from where it was before

Late Deceleration

(Most worrisome) Late onset of heart rate deceleration vs onset of contraction

Cause: Uteroplacental insufficiency

Treatment: Further testing

Repetitive and severe—emergency delivery

Treatment of moderate variable and late deceleration: Stop oxytocin, decrease uterine activity, correct hypotension; Give O_2 and fluid, change mother's position, perform vaginal exam to rule out prolapsed cord.

See Figure 13-8 for fetal heart rate graphs.

FIGURE 13-8 Example of Contraction Stress Test Showing Late Deceleration

(FHR) fetal heart rate in beats per minute

Uterine Contractions

Late Decelerations

PRETERM LABOR

Labor between 20 and 37 weeks
Treatment: Conservative, bed rest and tocolytics (B_2-agonist or Mg sulfate)

PROM

Premature rupture of membranes; rupture of membranes before onset of contractions
Increased risk of infection
Treatment:
> Preterm = bed rest and culture and Gram stain fluid
> At term, cervix favorable and no labor in 6–8 hrs = induce

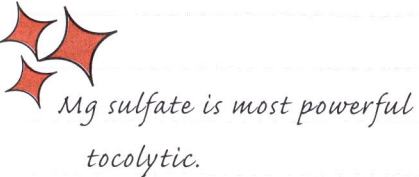

Mg sulfate is most powerful tocolytic.

Diagnosis of PROM:
Pooling amniotic fluid
Positive (blue) nitrazine paper
Ferning pattern on slide
Next step: U/S

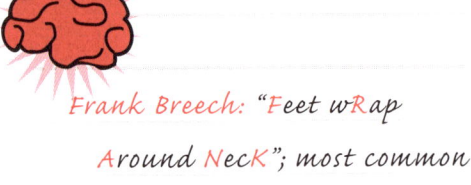

Frank Breech: "Feet wRap Around NecK"; most common fetal malpresentation

FETAL MALPRESENTATION

Frank Breech: "**F**eet w**R**ap **A**round Nec**K**"
Complete Breech: Knees and thighs flexed
Footling Breech: Extended leg(s)
Frank or complete breech *can* be delivered vaginally if: baby is small, at term, and both mother and fetus are healthy.
C-section must deliver footling breech.
Internal podalic version—twins.

POSTPARTUM HEMORRHAGE

> 1000 mL loss C-section
> 500 mL loss vaginal delivery

Uterine Atony
Most common cause of postpartum hemorrhage
Usually caused by *big uterus*: multiple gestation, polyhydramnios, macrosomia
Treatment: Uterine massage, oxytocin, methergine, prostin

POSTPARTUM FEVER

Most common cause is endometritis.
Other causes:
> UTI
> DVT
> Wound
> Mastitis
> Drugs

Treatment: IV antibiotics until patient is afebrile for 2 days

Endometritis
Occurs 2–3 days postpartum after prolonged labor, manual removal of placenta, artificial rupture of membranes
If does not improve after antibiotics—septic pelvic thrombophlebitis (treat with heparin)

Mastitis
Only seen in lactating women
Cause: *Staph aureus*
Treatment: Antibiotics and continue breast feeding

HIV mother should not breast feed.

CHAPTER 14 PEDIATRICS

Pediatrics is a highly tested discipline on the exam. Most review books provide much smaller sections for peds and OB/GYN as opposed to surgery and internal medicine. The exam contains many peds questions, and it is a subject that is easily forgotten for those not especially interested in this field. When studying, consider peds equally as important as surgery or internal medicine.

There are many aspects of peds that can be easily memorized and that will get you several correct answers on the exam. The following topics are easy to memorize and *always* on the exam: Apgar, developmental milestones, Tanner stages of development, and immunizations.

APGAR SCORE

Apgar score is given at 1 and 5 minutes of age:

Very good: 8–10
Good: 5–7
Poor: 0–4

See Table 14-1 for characteristics considered in Apgar scoring.

Screen all newborns in all states for PKU, galactosemia, and hypothyroid.

TABLE 14-1 Characteristics for Apgar Scoring

Apgar Score	Poor	Good	Very good
Appearance	Blue body	Pink and blue body	Pink body
Pulse	Absent	< 100	> 100
Grimace	None	Grimace	Grimace and cough or cry
Activity	Limp	Limited extremity movement	Active movement
Respiration	None	Slow cry	Strong cry

DEVELOPMENTAL MILESTONES

Social smile: 4–8 weeks
Rolls onto back: 4 months
Rolls onto stomach: 5 months
Sits without support: 6 months

Pincer grasp: 9 months
3 cubes: 15 months
Walks alone: 15 months
4 cubes: 18 months
7 cubes: 24 months
Rides tricycle, copies circle, counts 3 objects: 3 years old
Copies cross, square, counts 4 objects: 4 years old
Failure to Thrive: Always look at trend on the growth curve; if development is just slow and the *curve is normal*, it is only constitutional delay.

TANNER STAGES OF DEVELOPMENT

See Table 14-2 for Tanner stages of development.

TABLE 14-2 Tanner Stages of Development

Female	Pubic Hair	Breast Development	Notes
1	None	Preadolescent	
2	Minimal on labia	Buds with areolar enlargement	Around 11 years old
3	Increased, dark and curly	Breast areolar enlargement, areola level with breast	Growth spurt around 12 years old
4	Adult hair but not on thighs	Areola forms 2-degree mound, continuous enlargement	Menarche
5	Adult quality and distribution	Areola skin = with breast, adult size and form	

Male	Pubic Hair	Penis	Scrotum/ Testes	Notes
1	None	Preteen	Preteen	
2	Minimal at base of penis	Slight enlargement	Testes enlargement, scrotal skin redness, coarsening	12 years old

Normal findings: Treatment is reassurance!

Normal Findings:

Enuresis: Normal until age 5

Encopresis: Normal until age 4

Gynecomastia

Irregular menses at onset

Acne

Breast assymetry

Treatment: Reassurance

TABLE 14-2 Tanner Stages of Development (continued)

Male	Pubic Hair	Penis	Scrotum/ Testes	Notes
3	Increased, dark and curly	Penile "growth spurt"	Increased size	Nocturnal emissions common
4	Adult hair but not on thighs	Increased length and width	Adult	Growth spurt at 14 years old, gynecomastia common, facial hair around 16 years old
5	Adult quality and distribution	Adult		

Zero is before puberty.

IMMUNIZATIONS

Immunizations constitute another high-yield subject on the test. Actually knowing the entire immunization schedule is not that important. The questions are more geared toward side effects and indications/contraindications for each vaccine. Many test prep books include immunization schedules filling half a page, which I consider unnecessary. See Table 14-3 for a condensed immunization schedule.

TABLE 14-3 Immunization Schedule

HBV, DTP, Hib, Polio, Pneumovax	2, 4, 6 Months
DTP, Hib, MMR, Pneumovax, Varicella	12–15 Months
DTP, Polio, MMR	4–6 Years

The following are *not* contraindications for immunizing a patient:

1. Mild acute illness
2. Currently on antibiotics
3. Family history of seizure or SIDS
4. Fever less than 105 degrees after DTP

MMR Side Effects

1–2 weeks after immunization

Baby will present with low-grade fever, rash, and parotid swelling.

Influenza A Vaccine

Cannot be taken if allergic to egg

Recommended for:

Health care workers

Patients older than 65, especially in care facilities

Pregnant women *(in second and third trimester only)*

Patients with hemoglobinopathies, renal dysfunction, diabetes, cardiovascular or pulmonary disease, and those who are immunocompromised

Pneumococcal Vaccine

T-cell independent B-cell response

Recommended for:

Patients with diabetes, renal dysfunction, asplenia (SCA), cardiovascular and pulmonary disease

Patients older than 65

In children younger than 2, give conjugate vaccine; standard (PPV) pneumo vaccine is ineffective.

Rules for Immunizing Patients

1. Immunize chronologically even if child is premature.
2. If immunization is delayed, give as many immunizations as possible.
   Example: Young child moves from third-world country with no immunization history: What should you give her? Answer: all of them! Pick the choice with the most vaccines listed.
3. If a scheduled immunization is missed, at the following visit don't start over; pick up where you left off.
4. Do not give oral polio vaccine (live) to immunocompromised patients or patients with HIV+ status; in fact, only killed (Salk) polio is recommended for everyone.

Memorize this information about immunizations; there will be several questions on this topic.

HIV+ patients may receive all other vaccines unless the patient is severely immunocompromised; in this case MMR should be omitted.

5. Pneumovax, H. flu B, meningococcal vaccines: the capsule serves as antigen.

6. Every adult should be immunized every 10 years for diphtheria and tetanus toxoid.

PULMONARY CONGENITAL MALFORMATIONS AND DISORDERS

Respiratory Problems of the Newborn

The following disease processes will all present similarly. Each one will show signs of respiratory distress, cyanosis, and hypoxia. Even if you don't remember the specifics of each one, you can easily derive the diagnosis from the chest X-ray. In terms of treatment, for each one the immediate concern is proper oxygenation.

NEONATAL RESPIRATORY DISTRESS SYNDROME (NRDS)

Pathophysiology: Surfactant is not produced until 36 weeks. Surfactant decreases the surface tension in the alveoli. Without it, the alveoli collapse (atelectasis). Obviously the baby cannot oxygenate properly; therefore you can logically guess what the signs and symptoms will be.

Presentation: Usually presents in the first two days of life with cyanosis, grunting, and rapid labored breathing.

Tests: *Exam questions will commonly mention the chest X-ray appearance for RDS because it is the most common method used for diagnosis.*

ABG: Will show hypercarbia and hypoxemia.

Chest X-Ray: "Ground glass" appearance or a granular pattern seen throughout both lungs.

Treatment: To prevent this disease, try to prevent premature delivery. Giving the mother corticosteroids before delivery can help increase surfactant production in the newborn. You can monitor whether or not the baby is producing surfactant by checking the lecithin/sphingomyelin ratio. If the mother is diabetic, check the level of phosphotidylglycerol.

If premature delivery is inevitable, treatment is as follows:

Continuous positive airway pressure (CPAP)
Artificial surfactant

This is the most common respiratory problem in premature infants (commonly 28–30 weeks).

If these are not options in the answer choice, pick intubation and mechanical ventilation. Mechanical ventilation has a higher risk of complications vs CPAP.

Common Complications: Retinopathy of prematurity, pneumothorax, bronchopulmonary dysplasia, intraventricular hemorrhage, persistent PDA

TRANSIENT TACHYPNEA OF THE NEWBORN

This can easily be distinguished from RDS. It is usually seen after a **full-term** pregnancy with a **C-section** delivery.

Pathophysiology: The newborn has a small amount of amniotic fluid that remains in the lungs.

Test: Chest X-ray may appear normal (but don't let this make you miss the diagnosis!) or it may show *streaking* in the interlobular fissures.

Treatment: This is not nearly as serious as RDS. If hypoxic, give oxygen and it will resolve itself in approximately 3 days.

MECONIUM ASPIRATION

The newborn aspirates meconium; this diagnosis will seem evident in the exam question when they discuss the delivery. The baby will be hypoxic.

Tests: Chest X-ray will show patchy, coarse, or irregular infiltrates; may also see pneumothorax.

Treatment: Good suction, mechanical ventilation

Common Complication: Pneumothorax

DIAPHRAGMATIC HERNIA

This newborn will show signs of respiratory distress and a scaphoid abdomen directly after birth.

Pathophysiology: Congenital malformation of diaphragm that allows bowel to herniate into the chest causing an underdeveloped lung. It almost always occurs on the left side (Bochdalek).

Tests:
U/S in utero.
Bowel sounds will be heard in the chest on affected side.
Chest X-ray will show bowel in the chest.

Treatment: Surgery

In older child with respiratory distress, always consider aspiration:

Standing—right bronchi in superior segment of lower lobe

Supine or epileptics—posterior segment of lower lobe

GI CONGENITAL MALFORMATIONS AND PROBLEMS

Duodenal Atresia
Presents with bilious vomiting after each feed.
Increased incidence in **Down's syndrome.**
Test: Abdominal X-ray will show **"double bubble"** (air in duodenum and stomach).
Treatment: Surgery

Omphacele
Contains a sac; abdominal contents herniated through umbilicus
Treatment: C-section to prevent sac rupture and surgery

Gastroschisis
No sac; intestine herniates through abdominal wall, lateral to umbilicus
Treatment: Surgery

Anal Atresia
Detected early by exam in nursery

Choanal Atresia
Cyanosis (blue) when feeding; "pinks up" again with crying.
Child otherwise appears normal.
Test: (Diagnostic) inability to pass nasogastric tube

Tracheoesophageal Fistula
Blind pouch esophagus with distal esophagus connected to trachea. (There are other types but this is the only one that will appear on the test.)
From this description it is easy to imagine the presentation—polyhydramnios in utero, air in stomach, risk of aspiration.
TE fistula is commonly associated with cardiac and other anomalies.

VACTERL
Presentation: Coughing and choking with each feeding
Tests: (Diagnostic) Passage of NG tube with chest X-ray. You may also see aspiration on chest X-ray, but this is not diagnostic.
Treatment: Surgery

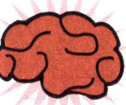

Congenital malformations = DOG

- **D**uodenal atresia
- **O**mphacele
- **G**astroschisis

These three always present early with polyhydramnios.

Umbilical hernia at birth is considered a normal variant and will close on its own by age 5. No surgery!

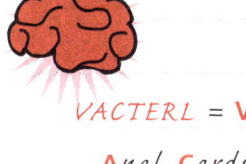

VACTERL = **V**ertebral, **A**nal, **C**ardiac, **T**racheal, **E**sophageal, **R**enal, **L**imb

Pyloric Stenosis

Easy diagnosis! More common in first-born males.

Presentation: Nonbilious, *projectile* **vomiting**, with palpable **"olive-shaped"** mass in abdomen

Tests: (Diagnostic) U/S will show hypertrophic pylorus; it may be referred to in the question as bird beak or string sign.

Labs Will Show: Hypochloremic, hypokalemic metabolic alkalosis

Treatment:

First: Correct electrolyte abnormalities! (Think logically—you would not take a child into an elective surgery with an electrolyte derangement.)

Second: Surgical correction (pyloromyotomy).

Intussusception

Telescoping bowel, age 0–2.

It is the most common cause of bowel obstruction, although it most commonly presents at 16–18 months of age.

Presentation: Crampy or colicky abdominal pain with sudden onset

"Sausage-shaped" right upper quadrant mass

"Currant jelly" stool

Diagnosis and Treatment: Barium enema (shows "coilspring" sign)

Meckel's Diverticulum

Presentation: **Pain*less*** rectal bleeding; this may cause intussusception

Test: (Diagnostic) Technetium scan

Hirschsprung's Disease

This is also know as *congenital aganglionic megacolon*. Intestinal obstruction results from no peristalsis or relaxation due to no autonomic innervation.

Presentation: Failure to pass *meconium*, bilious vomiting, intestinal obstruction, obstipation (no passage of bowel movements); also always consider cystic fibrosis with failure to pass meconium.

Tests: Barium enema shows dilated "megacolon" and narrow segments; (diagnostic) aganglionosis on rectal biopsy

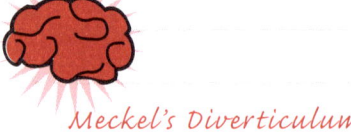

Meckel's Diverticulum:

Remember the rule of 2s?

2% of population

2 years of age

2 types of tissue

2 feet from ileocecal valve

Jaundice

Jaundice is pathologic or physiologic.

Tests (for both): Serum bilirubin (conjugated and unconjugated)

To Find the Cause: Coombs and Rh (mother and baby) and Hb

Physiologic Jaundice: (indirect or unconjugated) appears *after* 24 hours

Bilirubin peaks at 12.9 in 72 hours and resolves in 1 week.

Treatment: (Most commonly) Phototherapy or exchange transfusion

BILIARY ATRESIA

Elevated direct or conjugated hyperbilirubinemia

Presentation: Jaundice and clay-colored stool

Direct or conjugated hyperbilirubinemia is always pathologic. It is worrisome because it can lead to kernicterus.

Necrotizing Enterocolitis

This is a highly tested topic because it is *most common in premature infants.* (I am sure you remember this from the NICU.) It presents after the onset of feeding within the first 2 weeks of life. These babies also commonly have low Apgar scores.

Presentation: Lethargy, bloody stools, abdominal distension

Tests: (Diagnostic) Abdominal X-ray will show air in the bowel; WBCs are commonly elevated.

Treatment: NPO, antibiotics, decompression

If bowel becomes necrotic, surgical intervention is needed.

Diarrhea

Acute diarrhea in infants and children is either infectious in nature or caused by antibiotics.

For additional information, refer to Chapter 10, "Infectious Disease."

VIRAL

Rotavirus: The most common cause of diarrhea in pediatrics!

Test: Immunoassay

Treatment: Supportive

PROTOZOA AND ANTIBIOTICS

Giardia lamblia

Causes watery diarrhea with abdominal distension and weight loss. It is caused by cyst ingestion from contaminated food or water.

Commonly seen with drinking stream or well water while camping.
Steathorrhea plus protozoal cysts in stool.
Test: (Diagnostic) Duodenal aspirate

Entamoeba Histolytica
Causes bloody diarrhea and affects the colon.
May have a long incubation period of up to 3 months.
May mimic inflammatory bowel disease.
Tests: Stool culture, serology, biopsy

Clostridium Difficile
This is only seen after prior antibiotic use.
Example: Child plus infection plus antibiotic therapy plus diarrhea = clostridium
Tests: C-diff toxin in stool (*cytotoxin assay*); flexible sigmoidoscopy shows pseudomembranes
Treatment: For all three protozoa, metronidazole

BACTERIAL
For all bacterial causes you will see fecal RBCs and WBCs; therefore this is not diagnostic. Pay attention to other clues in the question.

Campylobacter
Most common cause of infectious diarrhea
Spread via contaminated food or water
Example: Ulcerative colitis–like symptoms plus *arthritis* = campylobacter
Treatment: Supportive, self-limited

Yersenia
Transmitted by contaminated food or animals
Example: Child with acute onset RLQ pain (like appendicitis) plus diarrhea = yersenia
Tests: (Diagnostic) Serology or stool culture

Shigella
Extremely contagious, person-to-person spread or from foods
Usually seen in **institutionalized patients** or **day care centers**
Commonly causes febrile seizures in young children
Example: Day care outbreak plus child with diarrhea plus new onset seizure = shigella
Treatment: TMP-SMX

Cryptosporidium can also cause diarrhea but is almost exclusively seen in the immunocompromised.

Salmonella

Spread through poultry, eggs, and milk

Associated headache, fever, malaise

Treatment: Supportive; antibiotics will prolong carrier
state

Enterotoxigenic E. coli

"Traveler's diarrhea"

Very watery diarrhea with no blood or fever

Treatment: TMP-SMX and loperamide

Enterohemorrhagic E. coli (0157:H7)

This causes diarrhea and HUS.

Example: Child with diarrhea later develops hemolysis,
uremia, thrombocytopenia.

Treatment: Supportive

Exam favorite! Remember the
highly publicized case with
Jack in the Box?

Lower GI Bleeding in the Neonate

This is most commonly caused by swallowed maternal
blood.

Test: Heme-positive stool

Diagnostic Tests: Apt test

Inflammatory Bowel Disease: Ulcerative Colitis and Crohn's Disease

For more information, refer to Chapter 7,
"Gastrointestinal."

Age of Onset: Adolescence

Presentation: Abdominal pain, fever, bloody diarrhea

Duration: Life-long, but patients experience remissions

Tests: (Diagnostic) Endoscopy and biopsy

Treatment: For both, steroids

ULCERATIVE COLITIS

Occurs only in the colon

Continuous lesions; involves mucosa only; commonly
associated with anemia

CROHN'S

Can occur anywhere in the GI tract.

Erythema nodosum; abscesses; fistulas; fissures; skip
lesions; granulomatous inflammation gives affected
area cobblestone appearance.

Gastroesophageal Reflux Disease in Children

As in adults, GERD is caused by relaxation of the lower esophageal sphincter. It is commonly associated with hiatal hernias. Presentation will be different in children. Obviously, a baby is not going to complain of heartburn.

Presentation: Apnea, frequent spitting up, possible vomiting plus poor weight gain and failure to thrive

Tests: (Diagnostic) pH probe; barium swallow

Treatment: PPIs, H2 blockers, antacids, prokinetics

GENITALIA

Hypospadias

Most common congenital malformation: Urethral opening on ventral side of penis

Presents as curved penis

Treatment: Surgical repair

Undescended Testes

Observation for 1 year to see if they come down on their own; if not, surgery

CONGENITAL HEART DEFECTS

Atrial Septal Defect

Fixed splitting of S2

Presents late in childhood/early adulthood

ECG: Right axis deviation

Diagnostic: Echo with color flow Doppler

Treatment: Antibiotic prophylaxis and surgery if over 2:1 ratio pulmonary to systemic blood flow

Ventricular Septal Defect

Most common congenital heart defect

Asymptomatic at birth

Pansystolic murmur, left lower sternal border, loud S2

Diagnostic: Echo

Patent Ductus Arteriosus

Wide pulse pressure, bounding peripheral pulses

"Machinery murmur"

Evaluation: Color flow Doppler

Treatment: Indomethacin unless *necessary* for survival (e.g., transposition of vessels)

Circumcision is contraindicated because it will block the opening of the urethra.

Undescended testes carry increased risk of testicular CA even after surgical intervention.

Most VSD close on their own! Treatment is reassurance.

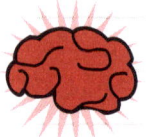

You can remember this by Police Department (PD) carries Machine guns.

Coarctation of the Aorta
Increased blood pressure in upper extremities vs lower
    extremities, rib notching
Diagnostic: Cardiac catheterization
Treatment: Cardiac catheterization or balloon angio

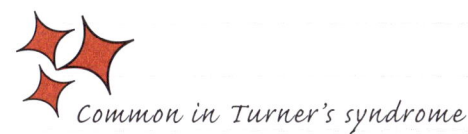

Common in Turner's syndrome

Transposition of Great Vessels
Most common cyanotic heart disease
Evaluation: Chest X-ray will show "egg on a string" heart
Treatment: PGE1 to keep PDA surgery

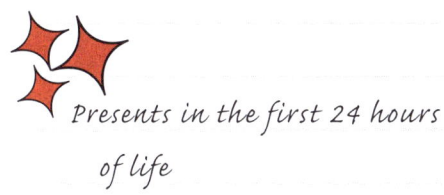

*Presents in the first 24 hours
of life*

Tricuspid Atresia
Cyanotic, presents early with left axis deviation
Evaluation: Chest X-ray will show snowman or figure eight

Tetralogy of Fallot
Most common cyanotic heart disease of childhood
Evaluation: Echo
Chest X-Ray: Boot-shaped heart
ECG: Right axis deviation
Treatment: Give PGE1 to keep the PDA open until surgery
Components: Pulmonary stenosis, overriding aorta, VSD,
    right ventricular hypertrophy
Complications: Ischemia, brain abscess, cerebral thrombosis

ONCOLOGY

Wilm's Tumor
Survival is over 90%; chromosome 11, from metanephros.
Most common renal tumor in children. Commonly
    associated with WAGR syndrome (Wilms, aniridia
    [no iris], genitourinary abnormalities, retardation),
    neurofibromatosis, Beckwith-Wiedemann syndrome
    (visceromegaly, macroglossia, hypertrophy).
Presentation: Most commonly presents as *mother finding
    painless lateral abdominal mass* plus microscopic
    hematuria, fever, hypertension.
Diagnostic Test: Abdominal U/S or CT shows intrarenal mass
    that distorts renal outline.
Treatment: Surgical removal plus chemo.

*The most common childhood
    CA is ALL!*

Retinoblastoma
Child with white reflex in eye instead of red

Commonly associated with

Down's syndrome

Neuroblastoma

Survival is around 80%; N-myc oncogene, amplification is bad prognosis.

Can present *anywhere* in neural crest.

Commonly presents as midline abdominal mass, hypertension.

Diagnostic Test: Increased catecholamines in urine, abdominal CT

CNS Tumors

Most common solid tumor in peds.

Most commonly found in posterior fossa, infratentorial.

Cerebellar Astrocytoma: Morning headache and vomiting.

Supratentorial: Craniopharyngioma causes short stature.

X-Ray: Large U-shaped sella.

ALL

80% of all childhood leukemias

Peak Age: 3–5 years old

Presentation: Thrombocytopenia, anemia, neutropenia

Diagnostic Tests: Bone marrow biopsy shows increased lymphoblasts

Bone Tumors

Common during periods of rapid growth

Ewing's Sarcoma: Onionskin appearance on X-ray

Osteosarcoma: Bone sclerosis on X-ray, increased risk of bilateral retinoblastoma

Neurofibromatosis

Cx 17, "Von Recklinghausen"

Most Commonly Presents As: hearing problems due to acoustic neuroma, Lisch nodules, and café au lait spots

   Prepubertal: 5 or more 5 mm in size

   Pubertal: 6 or more 15 mm in size

NEUROFIBROMATOSIS TYPE 2

Cx 22, bilateral acoustic neuromas

Diagnostic Test: MRI with gadolinium

Tuberous Sclerosis

Ash leaf spot (hypopigmented) and sebaceous adenomas, seizures

Diagnostic Test: CT shows calcified periventricular tubers

Sturge-Weber
Port wine stain, facial nevus, seizures
Diagnostic Tests: CT or MRI show intracranial calcifications

PEDIATRIC SEIZURES

For more information about seizures, refer to Chapter 12, "Neurology."

Febrile Seizures
Caused by rapid rise in body temperature in children (18 months–2 years old)
Generalized seizure for 10–15 minutes
Diagnostic Test: *Normal* EEG
Treatment: Bring down fever, *do not* give anticonvulsants.

Infantile Spasms (West Syndrome)
Peak Age: 3–12 months
Presentation: Tend to occur while drowsy or awakening; patient usually has multiple seizures per day
Diagnostic Test: EEG—Hypsarrhythmia, high amplitude/ slow wave
Treatment: ACTH, prednisone

Absence Seizure (Petit Mal)
10–30 seconds of LOC
Diagnostic Test: 3 per second spike and wave
Treatment: Ethosuximide

IMMUNOLOGY, GENETICS, ALLERGIES

Autosomal Recessive Diseases: 2/3 carrier, 1/4 affected
- Cystic fibrosis
- Albinism
- Alpha 1 antitrypsin deficiency
- PKU
- Thalassemia
- Sickle cell anemia
- Glycogen storage disease
- Mucopolysaccharidoses
- Sphingolipidoses
- Infantile polycystic kidney disease
- Primary hemochromatosis

X-Linked Recessive Diseases

Fragile X

DMD

Hemophilia

Bruton's agammaglobulinemia

G6PD

Lesch-Nyhan

Hunter's

Ocular albinism

Fabry's

Wiskott-Aldrich

Trinucleotide Repeat Diseases

Huntington's

Fragile X

Prader-Willi

Myotonic dystrophy

Frederick's ataxia

Lysosomal Storage Diseases

See Table 14-4 for a list of lysosomal storage diseases and their major characteristics.

TABLE 14-4 Lysosomal Storage Diseases

	Disease	Enzyme	Characteristics
XR	Fabry's	Alpha galactosidase A	Corneal clouding, cataracts, early renal failure
XR	Hunter's	Iduronate sulfatase	Mild retardation
AR	Hurler's	Alpha-L-induronase	Retardation, corneal clouding, gargoyle facies
AR	Gaucher's	Beta-glucocerebrosidase	Crinkled paper macrophages, hepatosplenomegaly, Erlenmeyer flask legs, brain and bone marrow involvement, gargoyle facies, Ashkenazi Jews
AR	Tay-Sachs	Hexosaminidase A	Cherry-red macula, death by 3 years old, Ashkenazi Jews

TABLE 14-4 Lysosomal Storage Diseases (continued)

	Disease	Enzyme	Characteristics
AR	Niemann-Pick	Sphingomyelinase	Death by 3 years old, cherry-red macula, zebra bodies
AR	Sandhoff's	Hexosaminidase A and B	Cherry-red macula
AR	Krabbe's	Galactosylceramide beta galactosidase	Brain involvement, globoid bodies, optic atrophy, spasticity, early death
AR	Metachromatic leukodystrophy	Arylsulfatase A	Like multiple sclerosis in 5- to 10-year-olds Brain, liver, kidney, nerve involvement

Immunodeficiencies

B-cell disorders = increased risk for bacterial infection

T-cell disorders = increased risk for fungal, viral, protozoal infection

B-CELL

Bruton's Agammaglobulinemia (X-linked)
B-cell deficiency found exclusively in males

T-CELL

IgA Deficiency
Most common immunodeficiency, usually asymptomatic, usually presents itself with anaphylaxis after blood transfusion

DiGeorge Syndrome
Thymic aplasia, cleft palate, hypocalcemia, Cx 22

B- AND T-CELL

SCID
Presents with frequent viral, fungal, and bacterial infections

Wiskott-Aldrich Syndrome
Increased IgE, IgA; decreased IgM

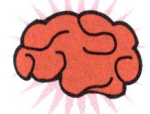

B-cell deficiency in Boys = increased risk for Bacterial infection

(XR) Thrombocytopenia, recurrent Infections, Excema "Wiskott wears a bow tie"

OTHER

C1 Esterase Deficiency
(AD) Angioedema (recurrent episodes of nonpitting
    edema), C4 complement is low
Treatment: Danazol

Terminal Complement Deficiency
(C5–C9) Recurrent meningococcal and gonococcal
    infections

Chronic Granulomatous Disease
Superoxide deficiency in macrophages
NBT+ (nitroblue tetrazolium test positive)

Chédiak-Higashi Syndrome
Defective neutrophil chemotaxis
Neutropenia, neuropathy, oculocutaneous albinism

Chronic Type I Hypersensitivity
Allergy, elevated IgE, eosinophilia
Asthma, allergic rhinitis, allergic shiners, nasal crease

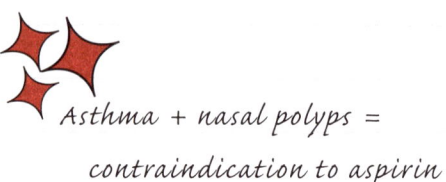

Asthma + nasal polyps =

contraindication to aspirin

Genetics

DOWN'S SYNDROME
Trisomy 21, most common cause of mental retardation
Increased risk with increased maternal age
Increased risk for duodenal atresia, ALL, early
    Alzheimer's disease

EDWARD'S SYNDROME
Trisomy 18, mental retardation plus overlapping
    fingers and clenched fist

PATAU'S SYNDROME
Trisomy 13, mental retardation plus rocker bottom feet

TURNER'S SYNDROME
XO, coarctation of aorta, rib notching on chest X-
    ray, amenorrhea, shield chest, wide-spaced nipple,
    webbed neck, kidney malformation

KLINEFELTER'S SYNDROME
XXY, tall, *infertility*, gynecomastia, microtestes

FRAGILE X SYNDROME

XR, second most common cause of mental retardation, large testes and jaw

PKU

Decreased PHE hydroxylase
Fair skin, musty odor, eczema
Treatment: Increase Tyr and decrease PHE in diet

Do not breast feed.

GALACTOSEMIA

AR, vomiting, jaundice, hypoglycemia, cataracts

SICKLE CELL ANEMIA

AR, signs and symptoms are not present until around 2 months of age (which is the time fetal hemoglobin decreases).
Dactylitis (infarcted fingers and toes commonly seen in infants), bone infarcts, pneumococcus and salmonella infections are very common.
Eventually the spleen will infarct.
Sickled cells and Howell-Jolly bodies are commonly seen on peripheral smear.
Diagnostic Test: Electrophoresis
Sickle Cell Trait: Most common presentation is painless hematuria.
Diagnostic Test: 40% on electrophoresis

HEMOPHILIA A

XR (factor 8 deficiency), most common presentation is hemarthrosis.
Treatment: Replace factor 8

LESCH–NYHAN

Self-mutilation and gouty arthritis

Fasciculations on tongue
(ocular muscles are spared)

WERDNIG HOFFMAN

AR, commonly presents as mentally normal floppy baby with frog-leg posture.
Tests: EMG will show fibrillations; muscle biopsy will show denervation; nerve conduction studies will show slow conduction.

DUCHENNE MUSCULAR DYSTROPHY

XR, most commonly presents as hip girdle weakness

Positive Gower's sign—child using hands to walk up legs in order to stand

Diagnostic Tests: Muscle biopsy; highly increased creatine kinase

CYSTIC FIBROSIS

AR, long arm of Cx 7

Presentation: Meconium ileus, recurrent URIs, and salty-tasting baby

Diagnostic Test: Sweat chloride test

HEREDITARY SPHEROCYTOSIS (AD)

Presentation: Jaundice and anemia

Diagnostic Test: Osmotic fragility test

Treatment: Splenectomy

PEDIATRIC INFECTIONS AND OTHER TIDBITS

Sepsis/Meningitis

Less than 1 month old (GEL)	Group B strep, *E. coli,* listeria
1–3 months	Pneumococci, meningococci
3 months–adult	Pneumococci, meningococci
Military/dormitory	Meningococci (petechiae)
Older than 60	Pneuomococci, G-bacilli, listeria

Encephalitis presents the same way but is more commonly caused by HSV, arbovirus, or pneumococcus.

SPECIFIC PRESENTATIONS

Encephalitis: *Confused*

Meningitis: Stiff neck plus photophobia

Abscess Alone: Focal deficit

In general CNS infections may present as: Fever, headache, nuchal rigidity

Upon Examination: Positive Kernig's, positive Brudzinski's

Focal neurological signs are possible.

Increased intracranial pressure (papilledema).

In babies, look for bulging fontanelle.

Do CT scan before LP if any signs of increased ICP!

Altered mental status.
Tests:
CT may show focal lesion.
If you need CT before LP, give patient ceftriaxone.
Tests: Culture is the best, most accurate, specific, etc.

CSF FINDINGS
Bacterial: Increased PMNs, decreased glucose,
    increased protein
Viral: Increased monocytes, normal glucose, normal or
    increased protein
Fungal: Increased monocytes, decreased glucose,
    normal or increased protein
Clues:
        India ink stain for cryptococcus
        Giemsa stain for trypanosomes
        PCR for herpes
        RBCs may be seen with HSV encephalitis
        CMV encephalitis if treated with gancyclovir and
            foscarnet
Treatment: HSV IV acyclovir; before culture comes
    back, if you suspect bacterial give vancomycin.
        Close contacts for meningococcus is rifampin
            (side effect: turns secretions orange).

Meningococcus always causes petechiae; therefore look for them in the presentation.

Guillain-Barre
Presentation: Ascending weakness after URI or other
    illness; lose deep tendon reflexes
Treatment: Plasmapheresis, IVIG, supportive

Congenital Hip Problems and Disorders
For types of congenital hip diseases and their treatment,
    see Table 14-5.

To contrast, botulism is a descending weakness and is usually seen in babies whose bottles are sweetened with honey or molasses.

TABLE 14-5 Congenital Hip Diseases and Treatment

Disease	Age	Features		Treatment
SCFE	9–13 years old	*Obese*	Knee/hip pain, also look for gonadal deficiency Test: LH, FSH, thyroid	Surgical pin
Legg-Calvé-Perthes	4–10 years old	Short boy with avascular necrosis of femoral head	Painless–painful Knee/hip pain	Orthoses
Congenital hip dysplasia	Birth–3 years old	Breech delivery	Ortolani's or Barlow's sign *Click* Diagnosis via U/S	Pavlik harness

Osgood–Schlatter

Physically active 10- to 15-year-old with *bilateral* knee pain and swelling of tibial tubercle

Scoliosis

Prepubescent girl with lateral curve of back

Neonatal Conjunctivitis

Easily distinguished by age; see Table 14-6 for details.

TABLE 14-6 Neonatal Conjunctivitis

Age	Treatment	Cause
First 24 hours	Chemical (caused by drops)	Observation, resolves within 2 days
2–5 days old	Gonorrhea	Erythromycin ointment
5–15 days	Chlamydia	Erythromycin drops and systemic due to risk of systemic infection

ToRCHeS

See Chapter 10, Table 10-9 for details on ToRCHeS.

AIRWAY ILLNESSES

Croup
Parainfluenza virus
Peak Age: 4–5 years old, usually in winter
Presentation: Inspiratory stridor, *barking cough*
Diagnostic Test: X-ray shows steeple sign
Treatment: Steroids and humidified air

Epiglottitis
H. influenza
Peak Age: 3–10 years old
Presentation: Muffled voice, *lean* forward and *drooling*, cherry-red epiglottis
Treatment: *Emergency*; take to OR and intubate immediately.
Test: Thumbprint sign on X-ray, but if you suspect this illness, don't wait for X-ray results to take action.

Pharyngitis
Group A strep
Diagnostic Test: Throat culture
Complications: GN, rheumatic fever

Retropharyngeal Abscess
High fever, drooling
Diagnostic Test: Lateral X-ray

Peritonsilar Abscess
High fever; bulging, swollen tonsils; and "hot potato" voice
Treatment: Culture abscess

Asthma
Reversible airway disease that is almost impossible to diagnose before 2 years old
Presentation: Wheezing
Treatment: (Acute) Bronchodilators and steroids

Rheumatic Fever
Cause is untreated strep throat; therefore, look for previous sore throat in question stem.
Most commonly affects mitral valve

Uvula deviates away from affected side.

Must have two or more from list of major criteria for rheumatic fever diagnosis:
Subcutaneous nodules
Polyarthritis
Erythema marginatum
Chorea
Carditis

OTHER CHILDHOOD ILLNESSES

Alport's Syndrome
(XD) Hearing loss, cataracts, and microscopic hematuria

Acute Glomerulonephritis
Look for recent sore throat in question stem
Presentation: Hypertension, hematuria, edema
Diagnostic Tests: RBC casts in urine, decreased C3 in blood
Treatment: Almost always supportive because the vast majority of cases resolve on their own

Nephrotic Syndrome
Look for history of URI symptoms
Edema, hyperlipidemia, hypoproteinemia, proteinuria
Diagnostic Tests: C3 is normal in blood; peritonitis may be seen, therefore expect a *very* sick patient.

Juvenile Rheumatoid Arthritis

THREE SUBTYPES
1. **Systemic:** Notice joint symptoms after appearance of salmon-colored rash and daily fever spikes
2. **Pauciarticular:** *Most common*; affects large joints only (weight-bearing joints)
   ANA Type: Iridiocyclitis plus asymmetric joint involvement
   RF Type: *Poor prognosis*; associated with Osgood-Schlatter (HLA-B27)
3. **Polyarticular:** Affects many small joints; most closely resembles adult RA without systemic symptoms

STILL'S DISEASE
Systemic juvenile rheumatoid arthritis with rash, high fever, knee pain
Labs: Leukocytosis, thrombocytosis with increased ESR
Treatment: Monitor LFTs and NSAIDs

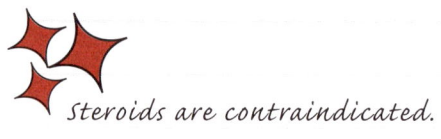
Steroids are contraindicated.

Kawasaki's Disease
Diagnosis is made from meeting 4 or more of the following criteria:
- Fever over 40° C for more than 5 days
- Conjunctivitis

- Rash
- Strawberry tongue
- Adenopathy
- Skin sloughing on hands and feet

Tests: Increased ESR and thrombocytosis
Treatment: Aspirin and IVIG

Ear Infections

OTITIS MEDIA

Strep pnuemo, H. flu
Bulging tympanic membranes, landmarks difficult to
    visualize
Treatment: Amoxicillin

OTITIS EXTERNA

Pseudomonas
Pain and discharge from canal in child who swims
Treatment: Ear drops

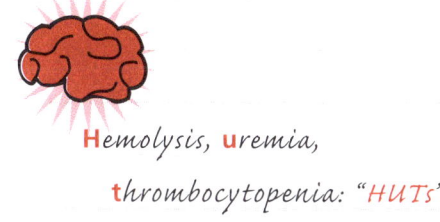

*Pain with movement of
external ear.*

INFECTIOUS MYRINGITIS

Mycoplasma, *strep pneumo*, virus
Vesicles on tympanic membrane

Viral Illnesses

For details on viral illnesses, see Chapter 10, Table 10-5.

Three-Letter Wonders

ITP

No fever, no splenomegaly, basically healthy with
    petechiae and purpura
Tests: Low platelets
Diagnostic: IgG test associated with platelets

HUS

Seen after food poisoning with *E. coli* 0157H7
Treatment: Supportive

TTP

Hemolysis, uremia, thrombocytopenia plus fever,
    confusion, splenomegaly
Treatment: Plasmapheresis

Hemolysis, **u**remia,
thrombocytopenia: *"HUTs"*

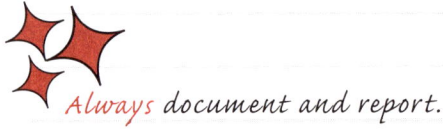

Always document and report.

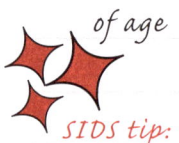

Most common cause of death from ages 1–12 months is SIDs. Peaks at 2–3 months of age

SIDS tip:

Always put babies to sleep on their backs.

Child Abuse Clues and Classic Presentations

- Large bite mark over 3 cm
- Old or healing fractures
- STD in young child
- Retinal hemorrhage due to shaking
- Bucket-handle fractures on X-ray
- Spiral fractures
- Subdural hematomas

Mortality

1. Motor vehicle accident
2. Suicide
3. Homicide
4. CA

See Table 14-7 for common pediatric poisonings.

TABLE 14-7 Common Pediatric Poisonings

Substance	Presentation	Antidote
Iron	Opacities on abdominal X-ray plus bloody diarrhea	Deforoxamine
Lead	Lead lines on X-ray	EDTA or BAL
Carbon monoxide	Cherry-red blood on ABG	Oxygen plus hyperbaric chamber
TCAs	Arrhythmia plus seizure (example: little boy has new onset seizure who has a brother who is on drugs for enuresis)	Alkalinize the urine
Aspirin	Metabolic acidosis with respiratory alkalosis	Aspirin ferric chloride test identifies exposure
Acetaminophen	Nausea and vomiting plus LFT derangement	N-acetylcystiene

CHAPTER 15 PREVENTIVE MEDICINE AND EPIDEMIOLOGY

ADULT VACCINATIONS

Adults should be immunized every 10 years for diphtheria and tetanus toxoid.

Capsules serve as antigen in vaccine (pneumovax, *H. influenza B.*, meningococcal).

Influenza A Vaccine

Contraindicated if allergic to eggs

Recommended for

- Patients 65 years old and older (especially in chronic care facilities)
- *Pregnant* women in second and third trimester
- Patients with cardio/pulmonary disease, DM, hemoglobinopathies, renal dysfunction, or who are immunocompromised
- Health care workers

Pneumococcal Vaccine

T-cell independent B-cell response

Recommended for

- Patients 65 years old and older
- Patients with cardio/pulmonary disease, DM, nephrotic syndrome, cirrhosis, asplenia

PPV 23: **Standard pneumococcal vaccine:** Not effective in children less than 2 years of age (instead administer the new conjugate vaccine)

For tetanus and immunizations in the immunocompromised patient, see Tables 15-1 and 15-2.

TABLE 15-1 Tetanus Immunization

History of Tetanus Immunization	Clean Wound	Dirty Wound
Fewer than 3 doses of tetanus toxoid in the past	TT: Yes TIG: No	TT: Yes TIG: No
3 or more doses of tetanus toxoid in the past	TT: Yes, if last dose was more than 10 years ago TIG: No	TT: Yes, if last dose was more than 5 years ago TIG: No

TT—tetanus toxoid; TIG—tetanus immunoglobulin

Measles and varicella vaccines are contraindicated in pregnant patients.

TABLE 15-2 Vaccinations in the Immunosuppressed Patient

	No/Moderate Immunosuppression	Severe Immunosuppression
DTP	Yes	Yes
OPV	No	No
IPV	Yes	Yes
MMR	Yes	No
Pneumococcal	Yes	Yes
Influenza	Yes	Yes

Rubella

All women of childbearing age who have no immunization history.

Contraindicated in pregnant women.

Women should avoid pregnancy for 3 months after receiving vaccine.

Contraindicated in immunocompromised patients *except* HIV patients.

HIV patients should receive the vaccine.

Health care workers should receive the vaccine.

Hepatitis B

Give to anyone at risk of contracting (e.g., health care workers) and anyone who wants it.

Immunizations in HIV+ Patients: If patient does not have severe immunosuppression, can give MMR.

REPORTABLE DISEASES

Required to Report to the CDC: Salmonella, shigella, coccidioidmycosis, cryptosporidiosis, viral hepatitis, TB, Lyme disease, cholera, varicella, HIV, AIDS, syphilis, gonorrhea, chlamydia, measles, mumps, rubella, diphtheria, tetanus, pertussis

DISEASE PREVENTION

Primary Prevention: Reduce the development of disease through health-promoting measures

Secondary Prevention: Early detection when mild or asymptomatic

Tertiary Prevention: Decrease morbidity associated with disease

EPIDEMIOLOGY

Per-year rates used to compare groups

Birth Rate: Live births/1000 population

Death Rate: Deaths/1000 population

Fertility Rate: Live births/1000 population of 15- to 45-year-old women

Neonatal Mortality Rate: Neonatal deaths (in first 28 days)/1000 live births

Perinatal Mortality Rate: Stillbirths/1000 total births plus neonatal deaths

Infant Mortality Rate: Deaths (age 0–1 year old)/1000 live births

Maternal Mortality Rate: Maternal pregnancy-related deaths (during pregnancy or up to 42 days after delivery)/100,000 live births

For cancer occurrence and cancer deaths, see Table 15-3; for leading causes of death by age, see Table 15-4; for cancer screening and other health screenings, see Tables 15-5 and 15-6.

TABLE 15-3 Cancer Incidence and Cancer Death

Most Common Incidence of Cancer		Most Common Cancer Deaths	
Male	**Female**	**Male**	**Female**
1. Prostate	Breast	1. Lung	Lung
2. Lung	Lung	2. Prostate	Breast
3. Colon	Colon	3. Colon	Colon

TABLE 15-4 Leading Causes of Death

Older than 60	Heart disease, lung cancer, CV disease, COPD, pneumonia, colorectal cancer
40–60 years old	Heart disease, breast cancer, lung cancer
13–39 years old	MVAs, suicide, homicide, injuries
7–12 years old	MVAs, injuries, leukemia, homicide
2–6 years old	Injuries, MVAs, congenital anomalies
Birth–18 months	Perinatal conditions, congenital anomalies, injuries

Lung cancer is the most common cause of cancer-related death in all groups except black females, for whom breast cancer deaths are more common.

TABLE 15-5 Cancer Screening

Skin exam	Self-exam every month Age 20–40: Every 3 years (by clinician) Older than 40: Annually (by clinician)
Mammography	Older than 40: Every 1–2 years Older than 50: Annually
Breast exam by clinician	Older than 40: Annually
Breast self-exam	Older than 20: Monthly
Pap smear	After 2 consecutive annual normal exams: every 3 years
Pelvic exam	Age 20–40: Every 3 years Older than 40: Annually
Prostate exam	Older than 50: Annually Older than 40: DRE annually
Flexible sigmoidoscopy	Older than 50: Every 5 years Older than 40: For high-risk patients

TABLE 15-6 Other Health Screenings in Addition to Cancer Screening

25–64 years old	BP every 2 years Cholesterol every 5 years Rubella serology or vaccination in women of childbearing age Alcohol abuse Depression
65 years old and older	Vision screening Hearing screening Alcohol abuse Depression

Screen for HCV if patient had blood transfusion before 1992.
Screen for HBV if patient had blood transfusion before 1986.

GOVERNMENT AND INSURANCE

Medicaid
Assistance for the indigent

Medicare
Health insurance for patients who are:
- Older than 65
- Permanently disabled
- Suffering from end-stage renal disease

ETHICAL AND LEGAL ISSUES

Disclosure
Full Disclosure: Patients have the right to know about their medical condition, prognosis, and treatment options.

A patient's family cannot require a doctor to withhold information from the patient.

A doctor can withhold information from a patient, but only if the doctor determines the knowledge would:
1. Harm the patient
2. Undermine informed decision-making capacity

Basically, do not withhold information from the patient if the family asks, but withhold information from the patient if it is the patient's wish.

Confidentiality
Do not tell anyone about the condition of your patient unless:
1. They are an authorized family member
2. They are colleagues directly involved in the patient's care and *need* to know

Break confidentiality only in the following situations:
- Suspected child abuse
- Court mandate
- Patient has a reportable disease
- Patient asks you to do so
- Patient states he or she is going to kill him or herself or someone else—report to authorities (Tarasoff decision)
- Patient is a danger to others (e.g., seizures or blind—report it to the DMV)

Informed Consent

Giving patient clear information about the:
- Diagnosis
- Prognosis
- Proposed treatment and treatment options
- Risk/benefit ratio

This information must be delivered such that the patient fully understands all parts.

Competency: Patients' authority to make their own personal and medical decisions

Decision-Making Capacity: Patients' ability to understand relevant information and refuse or accept treatment (determined by medical provider)

Treatment Refusal

Competent patients can refuse or stop treatment (e.g., don't force Jehovah's Witness to take blood products).

Incompetent, intoxicated, altered mental status (even clinically depressed patients) cannot refuse treatment.

Incompetent patients should have an acting surrogate decision maker appointed by the court.

Minors

Minors do not need parental consent in the following situations:
- Seeking drug treatment or counseling
- Seeking contraception, have an STD, or are pregnant
- Emancipated (serving in the armed services, parents of their own children, married, live on their own and are financially independent)
- Life-threatening situations (consent is implied)

CONFIDENTIALITY

You cannot break a minor's confidentiality even if their parent requests it.

Exceptions: Permission of the minor or if patients are a danger to themselves or others

CONSENT

Parents can refuse treatment for their children. If it is necessary, try to persuade the parent. The next option is to get a court order.

Precedent: In an emergency situation, if withholding treatment puts the child's well-being directly at risk, treatment can be started.

Parents may request their child be drug tested without their knowledge. This is unethical; do not do it.

Emergency situation involving a minor without parent present—treat as you see fit.

Written Advance Directives

Living Will: Expresses patient's wishes to withhold or withdraw treatment in event of terminal disease.

Examples: DNR/DNI—do not resuscitate/do not intubate does not mean do not treat; still administer all medical procedures except what is specified.

DPOA (Durable Power of Attorney): Appointed health care decision maker can be used if patient becomes incapacitated; more flexible than living will.

Without DPOA or living will, decisions should be made by (in order):

1. Close family member (spouse, parent, adult children, or siblings)
2. Friends
3. Personal physicians

In absence of living will or DPOA, if there is family disagreement about a medical decision, contact your hospital ethics committee; last resort is court order.

Withdrawal of Care: Withdrawing or withholding care "legally" means the same thing. Provide palliative treatment to relieve pain and suffering even if it hastens the patient's death.

Euthanasia and Physician-Assisted Suicide

Euthanasia: Giving lethal agent with the intent to relieve pain and suffering; this is unethical and *illegal*.

Physician-Assisted Suicide: Prescribing lethal agent that patient will self-administer to end his or her life; currently only legal in Oregon.

Malpractice

Civil suit under negligence where the burden of proof is "more likely than not" instead of "beyond a reasonable doubt."

Damage to a patient can be attributed to a doctor's negligence.

Living will always overrides DPOA. If there is a living will in place and patient does not wish to be on ventilator but family demands it, do not put the patient on ventilator. The idea is to carry out the expressed wishes of the patient.

CHAPTER 16 PSYCHIATRY

Psychiatry is an easy section on the test. Know the
    parameters for diagnosis, medications, and side effects.

PRINCIPLES OF DIAGNOSIS

Axis I: Clinical psychiatric disorders
Axis II: Personality and developmental disorders
Axis III: Medical conditions
Axis IV: Psychogenic stress (6-point scale)
Axis V: Global assessment functioning (90-point scale)

MOOD DISORDERS

Major Depressive Disorder
Female/Male (2:1)
Average Onset: Around 25 years old
Average Length of Episode: 4 months or longer
Average Recurrence Rate: Greater than 50%
Risk Increases With: Age, stress, chronic illness
Socioeconomic status and race are *not* risk factors.
Symptoms:

- **S**leep (increased or decreased)
- **I**nterest (anhedonia)
- **G**uilt
- **E**nergy (fatigue)
- **C**oncentration (decreased)
- **A**ppetite (hyperphagia or anorexia)
- **P**sychomotor (agitation or retardation)
- **S**uicidal ideation

Diagnostic Requirements: Five or more SIGECAPS symptoms
    plus depressed mood for a consecutive 2-week period

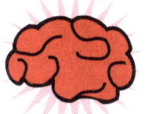

*Use "SIGECAPS" to remember
major depressive disorder
symptoms.*

Adjustment Disorder with Depressed Mood
Bad situation triggers depressed feeling for less than 6
    months, but criteria for full depression are not met.

Dysthymia
Depressed mood on most days for longer than 2 years
No episodes of hypomania, psychosis, or major depression

Treatments and Medications
Psychotherapy and antidepressants
    Anitidepressants may take 3 weeks to take effect and
        must treat for at least 6 months.

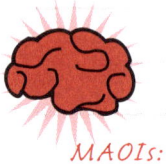

TCA overdose = cardiac

arrhythmia

Treatment = Bicarbonate

MAOIs:

PITS = Phenelzine,

Isocarboxazid,

Tranylcypromine, Selegiline

Don't be afraid to hospitalize

MDD patients because after

beginning meds, they will

have the energy to carry out

a suicide plan. Also, never

be afraid to ask patients

about thoughts of suicide!

ECT
Highly effective (usually 6–12 sessions)
Side Effect: Short-term memory loss

SSRIS (-OXETINES)
Prevent reuptake of serotonin
Side Effects: *Sexual dysfunction*, insomnia, anorexia

TCAS (-IPTYLINES, CLOMIPRAMINE)
Prevent reuptake of serotonin and NE
Side Effects: Sedation and *lower the seizure threshold*; block alpha-adrenergic receptors (orthostatic hypotension, falls, dizziness)

HETEROCYCLICS
Bupropion: First line for smoking cessation and depression
Side Effect: Substantially lower seizure threshold
Trazadone: Priapism is side effect.

MAOIS
Monoamine Oxidase Inhibitors
No longer a first-line treatment; good treatment for atypical depression (depression associated with hypersomnia or hyperphagia)
Side Effects: MAOIs plus tyramine-containing foods (wine, cheese, pâté) = hypertensive crisis
Serotonin syndrome is caused by taking MAOIs in conjunction with SSRIs or meperidine
Symptoms: Fever, myoclonus, cardiovascular collapse, mental status changes

Bipolar Disorder
History of mania alternating with depression is classic presentation, but mania is the only required symptom for diagnosis.
Average Age of Onset: 16–30 years old
Increased risk with family history
Mania Symptoms: Insomnia, increase in goal-oriented activity, delusions of grandeur, flight of ideas, pressured speech, poor judgment
- Bipolar I: At least one manic episode
- Bipolar II: Hypomania (does not interfere with occupation) plus major depression
- Cyclothymic: (Long term but less severe) 2 years of hypomania alternating with depressed mood
- Rapid cycling: 4 or more episodes in a year

Treatment:

First-line—lithium plus valproic acid (may cause liver dysfunction)

    Lithium: narrow therapeutic index (0.6–1.2 mEq); toxic (1.5–2.0 mEq)

    Side effects: tremor, nervousness, hypothyroidism, nephrotoxicity, diabetes insipidus

Second-line—olanzapine, gabapentin, carbamazepine (bone marrow depression), lamotrigine (life-threatening skin rash)

PSYCHOTIC DISORDERS

Schizophrenia

Caused by dopamine irregularities; increased risk with family history in first-degree relative

Age of Onset:

    Males: 15–25 years old (deteriorating male college freshman)

    Females: 25–35 years old

10% of schizophrenics commit suicide (past attempt best indicator of future success)

Diagnostic Criteria: Marked social and occupational dysfunction with symptoms for more than 6 months; see Table 16-1 for schizophrenia symptoms and prognostic factors.

TABLE 16-1 Schizophrenia Symptoms and Prognostic Factors

Positive Symptoms (Good Prognosis)	Negative Symptoms (Bad Prognosis)
Delusions	Flat affect
Bizarre behavior	Avolition (apathy)
Thought disorder	Alogia (no speech)
Decreased attention	Anhedonia

Good Prognostic Indicators	Bad Prognostic Indicators
Positive symptoms	Negative symptoms
Late onset	Early onset
Clear precipitating factor	No precipitating factor
Married/support system in place	Single/no support system
Family History: mood disorder	Family History: schizophrenia
Good premorbid function	Poor premorbid function

Time Period:
< 1 month = Acute/brief psychotic disorder
1–6 months = Schizophreniform disorder
> 6 months = Schizophrenia

SCHIZOAFFECTIVE DISORDER
Positive psychotic symptoms for 2 weeks
Meets criteria for schizophrenia and depression

SCHIZOPHRENIFORM DISORDER
Symptoms for less than 6 months

DELUSIONAL DISORDER
Nonbizarre delusions for 1 month or more
(No other symptoms)
Age of Onset: In 40s
Treatment: Psychotherapy

SCHIZOPHRENIA SUBTYPES
Paranoid: Delusions or hallucinations; no flat affect
Best prognosis
Catatonic: Two of the following—immobility, extreme
negativism, mutism, waxy flexibility, echolalia,
echopraxia, excess motor activity
Disorganized: Flat/inappropriate affect; disorganized
speech/affect
Worst prognosis

Antipsychotic Medications
There are two types of antipsychotic medications, typical
and atypical.

TYPICAL ANTIPSYCHOTICS
Block DA receptor (primarily D2)
High Potency: High incidence EPS (for EPS, see Table
16-2), low incidence of autonomic side effects,
works well on positive symptoms, works poorly on
negative symptoms
Low Potency: Less incidence EPS, associated with high
incidence autonomic side effects
High and Low Potency: Work well on positive
symptoms; work poorly on negative symptoms

Low Potency	**High Potency**
Chlorpromazine: Jaundice and photosensitivity	Haloperidol
Thioridazone: Retinal pigment deposits	Fluphenazine

TABLE 16-2 EPS: Extrapyramidal Side Effects

EPS	Time	Description	Treatment
Acute dystonia	4 hours	Muscle spasm, stiffness (torticollis, trismus), oculogyric crisis, tongue protrusion/ twisting	Treatment: Antihistamines (diphenhydramine) or anticholinergics (benztropine)
Akathisia	4 days	Feelings of restlessness; cannot sit still, constant pacing, sitting, standing	Beta-blockers
Dyskinesia (pseudo-parkinsonism)	4 weeks	Shuffling gait, masklike facies, stiffness, cogwheel rigidity *More common in older women	Antihistamines or anticholinergics
Tardive dyskinesia	4 months to 4 years	Perioral movement, involuntary choreoathetoid movements of head, trunk, and limbs 50% irreversible	Switch to newer psychotic; otherwise there is no treatment

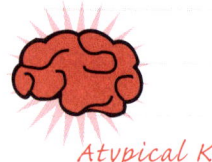

Atypical Key Words

Risperidone:

   Hyperprolactinemia

Olanzipine (also used to treat

   OCD)

Clozapine: Agranulocytosis

ATYPICAL ANTIPSYCHOTICS

Block serotonin and dopamine receptors
First-line (drug of choice) for maintenance therapy
Fewer extrapyramidal and anticholinergic side effects
Reduce negative symptoms
Side Effects Seen with All Atypical Antipsychotics: QT
   prolongation, weight gain, DM II

AUTONOMIC SIDE EFFECTS

(Anticholinergic) dry mouth/eyes, urinary retention,
   constipation, mydriasis, orthostatic hypotension
(Antihistamine) sedation

NEUROLEPTIC MALIGNANT SYNDROME

Can happen anytime while on antipsychotics
Fever, muscle rigidity, increased CPK, leukocytosis
Treatment: Stop causal agent; give dantrolene and IV
   fluids

ANXIETY DISORDERS

GAD (Generalized Anxiety Disorder)

Chronic, severe, obsessive worrying about multiple things
   at the same time
Twice as likely in females as in males
Age of Onset: Early 20s
Diagnostic Criteria:
   Worry on most days for 6 months or more
   Three or more somatic symptoms (sleep disturbance,
     fatigue, muscle tension, decreased concentration)
Treatment: First-line—SSRI or bupropion; second-line—
   benzodiazapine

OCD (Obsessive Compulsive Disorder)

Recurrent obsessions (thoughts or impulses) and
   compulsions (behaviors/acts) that cause great
   dysfunction of occupational or interpersonal lives
   Look for checking or washing rituals
Age of Onset: Adolescence/early adulthood
Diagnostic Criteria: Obsessions and/or compulsions that the
   patient recognizes as excessive and irrational; performs
   rituals for more than 1 hour per day
Treatment: SSRIs, clomipramine plus behavioral therapy
   (flooding technique)

PTSD (Posttraumatic Stress Disorder)

Patient who has experienced a life-threatening event and continues to relive it

Other Symptoms: Anhedonia, depression, survivor guilt, irritability

Diagnostic Criteria: Reexperiencing of the event and avoidance of stimuli associated with event for more than 1 month

Treatment: Group therapy, CBT, SSRIs

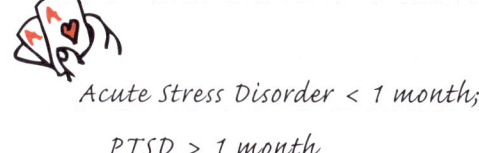

Acute Stress Disorder < 1 month;

PTSD > 1 month

Panic Disorder

Unexpected, recurrent panic attacks

Increased incidence of thyroid dysfunction and mitral valve prolapse

Panic Attack: Patients think they are dying with negative organic work-up for organic disease.

Commonly associated with agoraphobia (around 40%)

Diagnostic Criteria: Periods of intense discomfort/fear during which at least four of the following symptoms peak in 10 minutes: tachycardia, palpitations, chest pain, trembling, sweating, dizziness, fear of dying or going crazy; plus 1 month of concern of future attacks and/or behavioral change

Treatment: SSRIs

Social and Specific Phobias

Both types of phobias begin in childhood

Possible history of related events or panic attacks

SOCIAL PHOBIA

Marked anxiety brought on by social situations or performances (that cannot be avoided) in which embarrassment may occur—public speaking or social interaction

Treatment: B-blocker before event; behavioral therapy

SPECIFIC PHOBIA

Anxiety provoked by exposure to a feared situation/object (that cannot be avoided)—needles, blood, injection injury, animals, heights

Treatment: Behavioral therapy (systematic desensitization, flooding, biofeedback, etc.)

Dissociative Identity Disorder

Formerly known as **Multiple Personality Disorder**

Associated with childhood sexual abuse

Dissociative Fugue/Identity Disorder

Patient has amnesia and travels assuming a new identity—
  subconsciously with no malicious intent.

Homosexuality

Normal; *not* pathological at any age

Narcolepsy

Decreased REM sleep; genetic component

Bouts of daytime sleep (10 minutes–1 hour) plus cataplexy

Patients go to REM as soon as they fall asleep, cataplexy
  (loss of muscle tone), hypnopompic (waking) and/or
  hypnagogic (falling asleep) hallucinations

Treatment: Amphetamines and naps

Somatoform Disorders

Subconscious, unintentional, inappropriate behaviors

Treatment: Psychotherapy or frequent return visits

For somatoform, factitious, and malingering disorders, see
  Tables 16-3 and 16-4.

TABLE 16-3 "Faking It," Descriptions of Somatoform, Factitious, and Malingering Disorders

Disorder	Description
Somatoform	Symptoms created subconsciously (not intentional)
Factitious	Patients intentionally create their symptoms. Subject themselves to procedures in order to assume "patient's role" (no secondary gain)
Malingering	Patient intentionally creates illness for secondary gain (insurance money, etc.)

TABLE 16-4 Somatoform Disorders

Hypochondriasis	Believes has same disease despite recurrent negative work-up
Conversion disorder	Precipitating factor (relationship fight) followed by unexplainable neurological symptoms (blindness/numbness)
Somatization disorder	Many different complaints in many different organ systems over many years with extensive negative testing

Adjustment Disorders

Patient experiences depressed mood but does not meet full depression criteria.

For example, patient gets divorced and cries, stays in for a few weeks.

Personality Disorders

Lifelong disorders

Treatment: Psychotherapy

ANTISOCIAL

Almost always male.

Long criminal record, tortured animals, set fires as child.

History of conduct disorder is required for the diagnosis.

Shows no remorse or conscience.

Associated with alcoholism and drug abuse.

AVOIDANT

Inferiority complex; patient has no friends but does want them

Fear of rejection

BORDERLINE

"Splitting"; thinks people are all good or all bad

DEPENDENT

Patient cannot be or do anything alone; submissive; clingy

HISTRIONIC
Center of attention, seductive, overly dramatic

NARCISSISTIC
Egocentric; uses others for their own gain; lacks
  empathy

OBSESSIVE COMPULSIVE PERSONALITY
Inflexible rules, anal-retentive, restricted affect

PARANOID
Patient is distrustful, suspicious; thinks everyone is out
  to get them

SCHIZOID
Loner; no friends with no interest in having friends

SCHIZOTYPAL
No psychosis; strange, bizarre beliefs; "magical
  thinking"
Short psychotic episodes, unstable relationships

Gender Identity Disorder
More common in males.
Strong persistent discomfort with one's assigned sex
  without any underlying intersexual disorders.
Patient seeks surgical gender reassignment surgery.

Grief
After death of a loved one: numbness, bewilderment,
  distress, state of shock, sleep disturbances, crying,
  anorexia, decreased concentration, survivor guilt.
Symptoms are normal for up to 1 year.
Intense yearning and searching for deceased.
May have hallucinations/illusions but knows they are not
  real.
(Depressed patient believes they are real.)

ABUSE

Domestic Abuse
Male vs female
Pregnant women are at increased risk.
Many victims are eventually killed by their abusers.

Elderly Abuse
Usually live with their children, who are usually their abusers
Must be reported

Sexual Abuse
Abuser is often known to the victim, a family member, and male
Highest Incidence Age: 9–12 years old
Risk Factors: Single parent, substance abuse, crowded living conditions
Victim may exhibit genital or anal trauma, STDs, UTIs, and psychiatric complications.
All cases must be reported.

SUICIDE

Best predictor of future attempt: previous attempt
Risk Factors: Severe stress, family history, and schizophrenia
Greatest Risk Age Group: People older than 65
Third leading cause of death in 15- to 24-year-olds.
Always ask a patient about suicide.
Always watch for suicide in depression patients recently started on antidepressants.
Treatment: Ask directly about suicidal ideation, intent, plan, previous attempts, family history, hopelessness, ambivalence toward death.
If other treatments are refractory, consider ECT.

Women are more likely to attempt suicide.
Men are more likely to commit suicide.

If patient expresses desire or intent, hospitalize (even if involuntary).

EATING DISORDERS

Bulimia Nervosa
Peak Age: Late adolescence
Patients usually maintain normal body weight
Signs: Enamel erosion, scars on dorsum of hand
Diagnostic Criteria: Episodes of binge-eating out of control and purging 2 times per week for 3 months
More receptive to treatment than anorexia
Treatment: Psychotherapy and antidepressants if needed

Anorexia Nervosa
90% are female and commonly have a perfectionist personality.
Age of Onset: 15–30 years old
Patients exhibit restrictive behavior (fasting, excessive exercise).

Diagnostic Criteria for Anorexia
Distorted body image and intense fear of gaining weight
Body weight at least 15% below normal
Amenorrhea

DeliRIUM—change in sensoRIUM

DeMENtia—MEMory impairment

Mortality is greater than 10%.

Treatment: Psychotherapy, group therapy, antidepressants if needed

COGNITIVE DISORDERS

Delirium

Develops rapidly: hours–days and symptoms increase at night ("sundowning")

With or without hallucinations or illusions

Dementia

Diagnostic Criteria: Impaired memory and **one or more** symptoms increase at night ("sundowning")

For a comparison of dementia and delirium, see Table 16-5.

TABLE 16-5 Delirium vs Dementia

Delirium	
Age	Elderly, children, and hospitalized
Diagnostic criteria	Transient (temporary) disturbance in cognition and waxing & waning consciousness not due to dementia
Cause	Hypoxia, infection (UTI), meds, electrolyte derangement
Treatment	Treat underlying cause, optimize sensory environment Physical restraints if needed Low-dose anitpsychotic drugs for agitation
Dementia	
Age	Patients older than 85
Diagnostic criteria	Impaired memory and one or more of the following: agnosia, aphasia, apraxia, impaired planning with clear sensorium
Cause	Degenerative disease, endocrine, metabolic, exogenous (poisonings), neoplasia, trauma, infection, vascular (stroke)
Treatment	Low-dose antipsychotics Benzodiazepines are contraindicated.

SUBSTANCE ABUSE

Alcohol
Intoxication: Slurred speech, ataxia, hypoglycemia, retrograde amnesia (blackouts)
Withdrawal: Nausea, seizures, DTs, agitation, hallucinations, tremor

Marijuana
Intoxication: Impaired judgment, increased appetite, dry mouth, hallucinations, paranoia, conjunctival injections, amotivational syndrome

Cocaine
Intoxication: Insomnia, mydriasis, hypertension, sweating, hyperalertness, psychosis or "cocaine bugs"
Highly teratogenic (fetal vascular disruption)
Overdose: Possibly fatal—MI, seizure, stroke
Withdrawal: Crash—sleepy, hungry, irritable

Nicotine
Intoxication: Insomnia, restlessness, anxiety
Withdrawal: HA, cravings

Amphetamine
Intoxication: Hypertension, psychomotor agitation, insomnia, delusions/hallucinations, pupillary dilation
Withdrawal: Postuse crash HA, fatigue, hunger, depression

LSD and Mushrooms
Intoxication: Delusions, hallucinations, mydriasis
No withdrawal symptoms; patient may experience flashbacks months–years later
Treatment: Reassurance, antipsychotics, or benzos for bad trip

PCP
Intoxication: Agitation and aggressive behavior plus LSD symptoms
Vertical and/or horizontal nystagmus
Urine acidification will speed elimination
Overdose: Convulsions, coma
No withdrawal

Inhalants

Intoxication: Euphoria, dizziness, slurred speech, ataxia, sense of grandiosity

Most Common Users: 11- to 15-year-olds

Can cause permanent damage to CNS, liver, and kidneys

Overdose: Respiratory depression, arrhythmia

No withdrawal

Benzodiazepines

Intoxication: Sedation, drowsiness, reduced anxiety

Overdose (possibly fatal): Respiratory depression

Treatment: Flumazenil

Contraindicated with alcohol consumption

Withdrawal: Seizures; treat as inpatient with long-acting benzo and gradual tapering

Barbiturates

Intoxication: Respiratory depression

Withdrawal: Seizures

Opioids

Intoxication: CNS depression, seizure, nausea, vomiting, constipation, pupillary constriction

Treat Intoxication: Naloxone/naltrexone (block opioid receptor and reverse effects)

Withdrawal: (Can be fatal) anxiety, insomnia, piloerection, and nausea

Treat Withdrawal: Methadone (long-acting opioid)

PSYCHOLOGICAL TESTING

For a list of psychological tests and their descriptions, see Table 16-6.

TABLE 16-6 Psychological Testing

Test Name	Description
Beck Depression Inventory	Objective; depression screening test
Stanford-Binet	Objective; IQ test for adults
Wechsler Intelligence Scale	Objective; IQ for 4- to 17-year-olds

TABLE 16-6 Psychological Testing (continued)

Test Name	Description
Minnesota Multiphasic Personality Inventory	Objective; assesses personality type
Rorschach Test	Subjective; inkblot description
Luria-Nebraska Neuropsychological Battery	Assesses cognitive functions and cerebral dominance
Halstead-Reitan Battery	Detects specific brain lesion locations

Subjective: scored by tester; no right answer
Objective: scored by a computer

CHILD PSYCHIATRY

Encopresis
Not a disorder until after age 5; rule out physical problems
Treatment: Behavioral therapy

Enuresis
Not a disorder until after age 4; rule out physical problems
Treatment: Behavioral therapy; imipramine (refractory cases)

Mental Retardation
IQ less than 70 with adaptive function deficits
Onset before 18 years old
Number 1 preventable cause—fetal alcohol syndrome
Number 1 overall cause—Down's syndrome

Learning Difficulty
Academic functioning below average for age in reading, writing, or math
No mental retardation present
Rule out physical or social factors; remedial classes

Autistic Disorder
Symptoms evident before 3 years old; impaired communication and restricted activities
Stereotyped speech and behavior (hand-flapping)

Types of Mental Retardation
IQ Score (85% of cases are mild)
Mild 50–70
Moderate 35–49
Severe 20–34
Profound < 20

Childhood Disintegrative Disorder
Two or more years of normal development followed by severe developmental regression

Rett's Disorder
Genetic progressive disorder that affects females
Five months of normal development followed by progressive impairment

Tourette's Disorder
Multiple vocal or motor tics occurring multiple times per day consecutively for more than 1 year
Onset before 18 years old (around 20% utter obscenities)
Associated with OCD, learning disorders, ADHD
Remits during sleep and is exacerbated by stress
Stimulants precipitate tics
Treatment: Haloperidol, clonidine

Oppositional Defiant Disorder
Hostile, defiant behavior but does not seriously violate the rights of others
Misbehaves around adults but behaves normally around peers
Treatment: Family therapy

Conduct Disorder
Violating the basic rights of others, aggressive behavior, fire setting, cruelty to animals, stealing, fighting
More common in males with history of abuse
Some progress to antisocial disorder (after 18 years old)

Attention Deficit Hyperactivity Disorder
Presents between ages 3 and 13
Diagnostic Criteria: More than 6 symptoms for each category for more than 6 months in at least 2 settings before age 7 causing impairment
Inattention: Poor attention span, poor attention to detail, does not listen, easy distractibility, difficulty finishing tasks and following directions
Hyperactivity/Impulsivity: Fidgets, talks excessively, does not wait turn, interrupts others
Treatment: Methylphenidate or dextroamphetamine (may show reduced growth velocity)

Conduct disorder diagnosis as a child is required for antisocial disorder diagnosis as an adult.

CHAPTER 17 PULMONARY

ARDS

Noncardiogenic pulmonary edema caused by alveolar-
capillary membrane damage

Presentation and Diagnostic Criteria:

1. Acute onset respiratory distress
2. CXR—bilateral pulmonary infiltrates (pulmonary edema with normal heart size)
3. Severe hypoxemia ($PaFIO_2/FIO_2$ ratio < 200)
4. No evidence of cardiac origin (normal capillary wedge pressure 18mmHg)

Treatment:

1. Treat the underlying cause.
2. Correct hypoxemia.
3. Mechanical vent with PEEP
   Respiratory rate 12–20
   Volume 10cc/Kg
   Keep FIO_2 as low as possible.

See Chapter 14 for neonatal respiratory distress syndrome.

OBSTRUCTIVE LUNG DISEASE

For chronic bronchitis and emphysema, see Table 17-1.

TABLE 17-1 Precursors of COPD

	Cause	Diagnostic Criteria	Leads To
Chronic Bronchitis	Smoking	3 months with productive cough for 2 consecutive years	COPD
Emphysema	Smoking or alpha-1 antitrypsin deficiency	Pathologic diagnosis of airway destruction	COPD

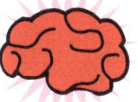

Risks with use of PEEP are diminished cardiac output and barotraumas.

Obstructive lung disease, can't get air Out.

FEV1/FVC < 80%
Increased TLC, FRC, RV
Decreased O_2 and pH, increased CO_2 and respiratory rate

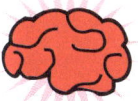

Obstructive lung disease is "COPD + BABE":

Bronchiectasis

Asthma

Bronchitis (chronic)

Emphysema

After quitting smoking, home oxygen therapy is the only modality proven to prolong survival in patients with COPD.

Physical exam is normal between attacks!

Cromolyn is only useful for prophylaxis; aminophylline is also not helpful in acute attack.

COPD

Presentation: Diminished breath sounds, increased AP diameter, corpulmonale (JVD, hepatomegaly, peripheral edema)
Diagnostic Tests: CXR shows flat diaphragm, hyperinflation, reduced vascular markings, bullae; polycythemia due to secondary hypoxemia; labs indicate respiratory acidosis
Treatment: Smoking cessation, bronchodilators, steroids, oxygen
COPD with collapsed lung—perform bronchoscopy and removal of mucous plug

ASTHMA

Reversible increased resistance to airflow due to airway bronchospasm and inflammation
Presentation: Coughing, wheezing, chest tightness
PE: Decreased breath sounds, accessory muscle use, wheezing
Trigger Factors: Exercise RTIs; cold or dry air GE reflux; airway irritants; aspirin/NSAIDs
Diagnostic Tests:
    PFTs—decreased 1s FEV1
    CXR—hyperinflation
    CBC—eosinophils
    ABG—hypoxia
    Respiratory alkalosis
Treatment: (Acute) Inhalers or systemic steroids, B2-agonists, anticholinergics

BRONCHIECTASIS

Permanent dilatation of bronchi
Usually follows RTI/pneumonia
Presentation: Rhales, wheezing
Diagnostic Tests: CXR—train-lines and honeycombing; CT—dilatation of airways
Treatment: Antibiotics, steroids, careful lung hygiene

CYSTIC FIBROSIS

Autosomal recessive disorder (chromosome 7) mostly seen in Caucasians

Presentation: Recurrent pulmonary infections, meconium ileus, rectal prolapse, malabsorption syndrome, abnormal GTT; staph aureus and pulmonary infections

Diagnostic Tests: Sweat chloride test > 60 mEq/L under 20 years old; sweat chloride test > 80 mEq/L in adulthood

Treatment: Fat-soluble vitamins, pancreatic enzymes, DNase, chest PT, bronchodilators, annual flu vaccine

PULMONARY EMBOLISM

Clot originates from deep veins, pelvis, or legs and lodges in circulation of lung

10% fatal

High PA pressure and may develop corpulmonale

Normal CXR

Presentation: Loud second heart sound, pleuritic chest pain, dyspnea

Risk Factors: Hypercoagulable states; BCPs; obesity; CHF; post-op patients, especially after leg or pelvic surgery

Hypercoagulable States: Strong family history and unusual sites of thrombosis (not leg or pelvis)

Causes: Antithrombin III; Protein C, S; malignancy, DIC, PRV, lupus anticoagulant

Diagnostic Tests: CXR—normal; ABG—hypoxemia, hypocapnia; increased arterial–alveolar O_2 difference; respiratory alkalosis

Treatment:

If thrombolysis is potentially fatal:

1. Heparin with target PTT 1.5–2.0
2. Then switch to warfarin target INR 2–3

No risk of DVT? Discontinue warfarin after 3–6 months.

Risk of DVT? Continue warfarin indefinitely.

Heparin

Enhances Antithrombin III

Monitor with PTT

Safe to give during pregnancy

Side Effects: Thrombocytopenia; antidote—protamine

Suspect PE?

1. Order V/Q scan.

Inconclusive?

2. Order venous U/S or CT angiogram of chest.

Inconclusive?

3. Order pulmonary angiogram (gold standard).

Warfarin

Vitamin K antagonist
Inhibits 2, 7, 9, 10 Protein C and S
Beware of P450 drug interactions
Teratogenic; contraindicated during pregnancy
Side Effects: Skin necrosis

Streptokinase, Urokinase, tPA

Stimulate fibrinolysis.
High risk of bleeding.
Use only with life-threatening PE.

Greenfield Filter

Use if patient can't be on an anticoagulant or suffers from
    recurrent PEs.

RESTRICTIVE LUNG DISEASE

Pulmonary fibrosis, pneumoconioses, sarcoidosis
Lung volumes are decreased
FEV1/FVC ratio near normal
Decreased O_2 and CO_2; increased pH and heart rate

DIFFUSE INTERSTITIAL PULMONARY FIBROSIS

Restrictive lung disease
Causes thick alveolar walls and dilated bronchioles
Drugs associated with interstitial lung disease—radiation,
    long-term vent, bleomycin, amiodarone, busulfan,
    nitrofurantoin
Presentation: Shallow, rapid breathing and nonproductive
    cough
Diagnostic Tests: CXR—honeycomb pattern; FEV1/FVC is
    increased (restrictive pattern)
Treatment: Supportive, cytotoxic agents, steroids

Other Drug-Induced Lung Disorders

Bleomycin—fibrosis
Amiodarone—pneumonitis with bilateral interstitial or
    alveolar pattern
ACE inhibitors—nonproductive cough
Narcotics—noncardiogenic pulmonary edema
IV drug users—septic emboli from right heart endocarditis
    (staph)

Hydralazine— drug-induced lupus (antihistone Ab)
INH—drug-induced lupus (antihistone Ab)
Procainamide— drug-induced lupus (antihistone Ab)
Ethosuximide— drug-induced lupus (antihistone Ab)
Beta-blockers—bronchoconstriction

PNEUMOCONIOSES

Occupational lung injury
Order CXR and confirm with CT

Berylliosis
Work in electronics, ceramic industries, die manufacturing,
    aerospace, electronics
Diagnostic Test: CXR—hilar adenopathy, infiltrates
Requires chronic steroid treatment

Coal Miner's Disease
Work in coal mines
Diagnostic Test: Small upper lung zone opacities

Silicosis
Work with silica, glass, or in quarries
Diagnostic Test: CXR—*eggshell calcifications*
Increased risk of TB

Asbestosis
Inhaled asbestos fibers cause pulmonary fibrosis reaction.
Diagnostic Tests: CXR—pleural plaques and thickening,
    hazy lower lobe infiltrates; biopsy—asbestos bodies
Increased risk of bronchogenic CA and mesothelioma

ALLERGIC BRONCHOPULMONARY ASPERGILLOSIS

Asthmalike symptoms
Increased IgE
Increased eosinophils
Central bronchiectasis
Positive Aspergillus shin test
Treatment: Prednisolone, itraconazole

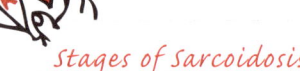

Stages of Sarcoidosis

0: Normal

1: Hilar lymphadenopathy

IIA: Hilar lymphadenopathy and parenchymal infiltrates

IIB: Infiltrates without hilar lymphadenopathy

III: Advanced fibrosis and bullae

SARCOIDOSIS

Chronic disease with noncaseating granulomas in affected organs

Most common in African American females

90% with pulmonary involvement

Presentation:

Skin—lupus pernio (blue-purple lesion of face and fingers)

Erythema nodosum

Nervous system—Bell's palsy

Eye—uveitis

Diagnostic Tests: CXR—bilateral hilar lymphadenopathy; histology—noncaseating granulomas; elevated ACE levels, hypercalcemia

Lofgren's Syndrome

Acute form of sarcoidosis with triad of ankle edema, erythema nodosum, and arthritis

WEGENER'S GRANULOMATOSIS

Nasal, lung, and kidney involvement

Presentation: Sinus infection, cough for 3–6 months, hemoptysis, hematuria, ARF

Diagnostic Tests: CXR—multinodular infiltrates; key labs— *elevated C-ANCA*

Treatment: Cyclophosphamide

GOODPASTURE'S DISEASE

Lung and kidney involvement

Diffuse alveolar hemorrhage and glomerulonephritis

Due to antiglomerular basement membrane Ab's

Presentation: Hemoptysis, dyspnea, hematuria, renal failure

Diagnostic Test: Linear immunoflourescence pattern on renal biopsy

Treatment: Steroids and cyclophosphamide

PNEUMONIA

Differentiate between typical and atypical bugs; see Table 17-2.

Diagnostic Tests: Elevated WBCs and CXR abnormalities

TABLE 17-2 Typical and Atypical Pneumonia

	Atypical Pneumonia	Typical Pneumonia
Age	Younger than 45	Older than 45
Fever	Lower than 102 degrees	Higher than 102 degrees
Prodrome	More than 3 days	Less than 2 days
CXR	Single lobe	Diffuse
Bug	Mycoplasma, Chlamydia, etc.	Strep pneumoniae
Medications	Azithromycin	Cephalosporins

In peds, multiple episodes of pneumonia (especially right middle or lower lobe) = foreign body aspiration

PLEURAL EFFUSION

Fluid accumulation in pleural space

Presentation: Pleuritic chest pain, dyspnea, cough; friction rub, decreased tactile fremitus, dullness to percussion, decreased breath sounds

Diagnostic Tests:

1. CXR: blunting costophrenic angle > 300cc; free-flowing fluid with lateral decubitus film.
2. Pleural fluid analysis: cell count/differential, chemistries, culture, stains, cytology.
3. Thoracocentesis is definitive and determines transudate or exudate.

Tube thoracostamy parapneumonic effusion when:

pH < 7.2

Glucose < 60

Infection

Transudate

Pleural/Serum LDH < 0.6

Pleural/Serum protein < 0.5

Causes: Protein-losing enteropathy, CHF, nephrotic syndrome, cirrhosis

Exudate

Pleural/Serum LDH > 0.6

Pleural/Serum protein > 0.5

Causes: TB, bacterial infection, malignancy, hemothorax, PE with infarct, pancreatitis, esophageal rupture

- Esophageal rupture or pancreatitis—increased amylase
- PE, TB, hemothorax— > 100,000 RBCs
- Infection—low glucose, high protein
- Empyema—frank pus in pleural space

Treatment of Both Transudate and Exudate
Hemothorax: Chest tube, treat underlying condition
Empyema: Chest tube drainage, thoracocentesis if dyspneic
Malignancy: Pleurodesis

PNEUMOTHORAX

Air in pleural space that can lead to collapsed lung
Presentation: Sudden onset of dyspnea, pleuritic chest pain, diminished breath sounds, decreased tactile fremitus
Diagnostic Test: CXR—lung retraction with best view at end of expiration
Treatment: Small—oxygen therapy; large—chest tube placement

Spontaneous Pneumothorax
Due to rupture of blebs
Secondary to COPD, asthma, bullous emphysema
Key Presentation: Young, thin, tall males

Tension Pnuemothorax
Medical emergency
Presentation: Loss of breath sounds on affected side with tracheal and heart sound shift
Treatment: Emergency chest tube!

SOLITARY PULMONARY NODULE

Single small node in lung parenchyma (< 6 cm); see Table 17-3 for benign vs malignant.

TABLE 17-3   Solitary Pulmonary Nodule (< 6 cm)

Favors Benign	Favors Malignant
Young	Old
Normal CXR	Smoker
Small (< 1 cm)	Large
Smooth margins	Eccentric calcifications

Presentation: Often asymptomatic (incidental finding on CXR or CT); otherwise—shortness of breath, cough, dyspnea

Diagnostic Tests:
   CXR (compare old and new)
   CT
   Bronchoscopy and biopsy
   Percutaneous needle biopsy
   Minithoracotamy
Treatment: If lesion has not changed in 2 years, follow-up study in 3–6 months; surgical resection for lesions that have changed

LUNG CANCER

Number 1 cause of cancer death
Presentation: Pneumonia that does not improve after 2 weeks with antibiotics
 With or without respiratory symptoms, paraneoplastic syndromes, Horner's syndrome
Risk Factors: Smoking and asbestos exposure
Diagnostic Tests: Same as nodule

Two Types of Lung Cancer
Non–Small Cell Cancer (NSCLC): Metastesizes less frequently than small cell cancer

Adenocarcinoma
Peripheral location

Squamous Cell Carcinoma
Central location, associated with hypercalcemia due to increased parathyroid hormone

Treatment:
NSCLC—IA, IB, IIA, IIB resectable; IIIB nonresectable

Small Cell Cancer (SCLC): Associated with paraneoplastic syndromes and may present as bone, brain, or liver METS

Treatment:
SCLC—not resectable

Paraneoplastic Syndromes
The following are seen with small cell carcinoma:
1. **SIADH:** Hyponatremic
2. **Cushing's Syndrome:** Hypertension, hypokalemia, hyperglycemia, proximal muscle weakness; no suppression with dexamethasone suppression test; hypercalcemia—bone METS or osteoclastic activity

3. **Eaton-Lambert Syndrome:** Myasthenia-like syndrome; muscle increase in strength with repetition; decreased DTRs; autonomic dysfunction

CHAPTER 18 GENITOURINARY/RENAL

BENIGN PROSTATIC HYPERPLASIA

Seen in men older than 50
Considered normal enlargement of the prostate with aging
Presentation: Urgency, frequency, urinary hesitancy, decreased force of stream, incomplete emptying
Urinary retention, UTIs, hydronephrosis
Diagnostic Tests: DRE—enlarged, rubbery texture
 Any detectable masses present = evaluate for prostate CA; screen for UTI and urinary obstruction
Treatment: Alpha-1 blockade (-zosins), 5-alpha-reductase inhibitors
    If severe with acute urinary retention, treat with transurethral resection of the prostate (TURP).

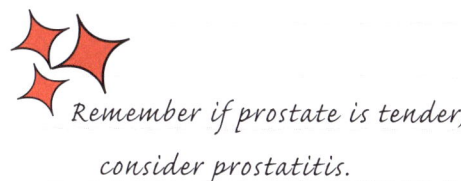

Remember if prostate is tender, consider prostatitis.

PROSTATE CANCER

Number 1 cause of cancer in men; number 2 cause of cancer deaths in men
Presentation: May be asymptomatic; or lymph edema, back pain, urinary retention symptoms
Diagnostic Tests:
    1. DRE—palpable nodule
    2. PSA: Elevated
    3. U/S guided transrectal biopsy (confirmatory)
Treatment:
    Low-grade tumors in elderly = watchful waiting
    Surgery plus radiation carries risk of incontinence and impotence
    METS present = treat with androgen ablation
Screening: Annual DRE for all men older than 50.
    Earlier screening for men with history in first-degree relative.
    PSA should not be considered a screening test.

ERECTILE DYSFUNCTION

Affects around 20% of older males.
Most commonly due to a vascular problem.
Patients rarely offer this kind of information, so inquire.
History often = diagnosis.
For causes, see Figure 18-1.

FIGURE 18-1 Erectile Dysfunction

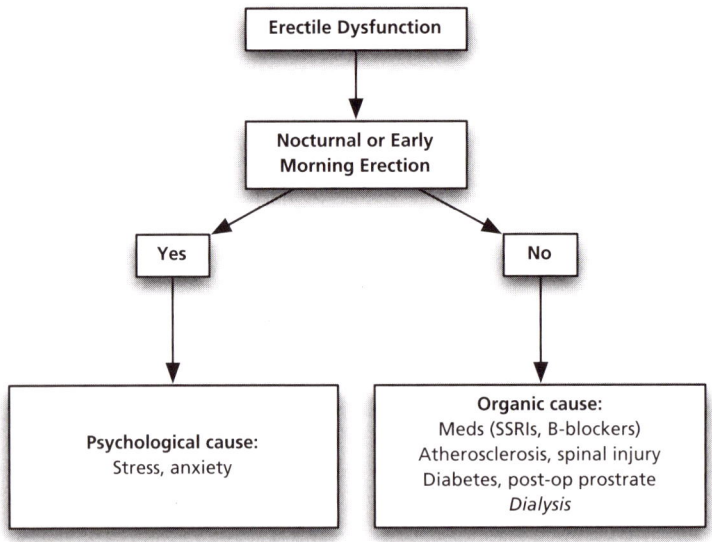

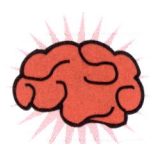

"Point and Shoot":

Parasympathetic mediates
erection, **S**ympathetic
mediates ejaculation

Treatment: (Psychological) Psycho- and/or sex therapy;
testosterone for patients with hypogonadism; sildenafil
for other causes

TESTICULAR CANCER

Men 20–35 years old
90% are germ cell (seminoma)
Presentation: Young man with painless mass
Main Risk Factor: Cryptochidism
Treatment: Radiation with or without orchiectomy
For testicular tumor markers, see Table 18-1.

TABLE 18-1 Testicular Tumor Markers

Alpha fetaprotein	Yolk sac tumor
HCG	Choliocarcinoma
Androgens with or without precocious puberty	Leydig cell tumor

BLADDER CANCER

Men 50–60 years old (transitional cell carcinoma)
Second most common urological cancer
Presentation: *Painless gross hematuria*
Tests: UA, IVP
    Cystoscopy plus biopsy are confirmatory.
Treatment:
    CIS and superficial CA: intravesicular chemo
    Distant METS: chemo only
    Invasive without METS: surgery with or without
      radiation

RENAL CELL CANCER

METS to lung and bone (adenocarcinoma)
Risk Factors: Smoking, male, Von Hippel-Lindau disease
Presentation: Hematuria with flank pain plus palpable
    mass
Commonly sends "cannonball METS" to lung
Treatment: Surgery

VON HIPPEL-LINDAU DISEASE

Increased risk of renal cell CA
Commonly associated with cysts in liver and/or kidney and
    cerebellar hemangioma

FANCONI'S SYNDROME

Carbonic anhydrase defect.
Lose amino acids, glucose, PO_4, calcium, and magnesium.
RBCs have no glucose and burst, causing Fanconi's
    anemia.

Always consider smokers and people who work in dye plants.

Bladder CA Risk Factors
- Smoking
- Schistosomiasis
- Aniline dyes (rubber and dye industries)
- Calculi

RCC:

Increased erythropoietin without hypoxia

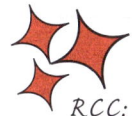

Embryology
Mesonephros—Wolffian duct
Paramesonephros—Müllerian duct
Metanephric—Renal
Allantois—Urachus-bladder

RENAL CALCULI

See Table 18-2 for the different types of renal stones.

TABLE 18-2 Renal Stones

Renal Stone Type	Frequency and X-Ray Findings	Characteristics
Calcium oxalate/phosphate	89%, most common Radiopaque	Hypercalciuria, hyperparathyroidism, alkaline urine
Struvite	7% Radiopaque	Possible cause:Infection Forms staghorn calculi
Uric acid	2.5% Radiolucent	History of gout or leukemia
Cysteine	1.5%, least common Radiopaque	AD—cystinuria Hexagonal crystals in urine

Nephrolithiasis

Risk Factors: Male, any condition that causes hypercalcemia, dehydration, gout, RTA

Presentation: Hematuria; severe, colicky flank pain with or without radiation to groin; patient moves around frequently and can't get comfortable.

Only uric acid stones do not show up on X-ray.

Too much vitamin C can cause Ca+ oxalate stones in patients with renal insufficiency.

Cystinuria is caused by defect in renal transport of cysteine, ornithine, lysine, and arginine.

    Diagnostic Test for Cystinuria: Cyanide nitroprusside test

Test: UA—hematuria, altered urine pH

Diagnostic Tests:

1. UA, KUB
2. Confirm with IVP

Treatment: *Hydration*, give narcotics until stone passes

Stone < 3 cm in diameter—lithotripsy

POLYCYSTIC KIDNEY DISEASE

Presentation: Large palpable kidney, pain and hematuria, HTN, berry aneurysms, hepatic cysts
Diagnostic Tests: U/S or CT
Treatment: Prevent UTIs, control HTN; ESRD—transplant
For the two types of polycystic kidney disease, see Figure 18-2.

FIGURE 18-2 PCKD—2 Types

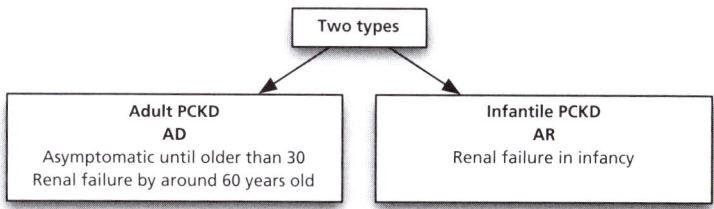

URINARY TRACT INFECTIONS

Much more common in females.
E. coli is causal agent majority of the time.
Presentation: Frequency, urgency, dysuria, suprapubic pain, fever
Test: UA—WBCs in urine, bacteria, positive leukocyte esterase, positive nitrite
Definitive Test: Urine culture, clean catch midstream sample
Treatment: TMP-SMX, amoxicillin, first-generation cephalosporins
For further information, see Chapter 13, "Obstetrics," and Chapter 14, "Pediatrics."

NEPHRITIC VS NEPHROTIC SYNDROME

Nephritic Syndrome
Hypertension, hematuria, oliguria, mild proteinuria; see Table 18-3.
Labs: Rising BUN/Cr
Key: RBC casts in urine

TABLE 18-3 Nephritic Syndrome

Poststreptococcal glomerulonephritis (PSGN)	Cause: Recent strep infection (Group A beta hemolytic)	IF: Lumpy, bumpy RBCs or RBC casts in urine Decreased C3, increased ASO No treatment
Wegener's granulomatosis Rapidly progressive glomerulonephritis	Respiratory tract inflammation plus necrotizing vasculitis	Sinus symptoms and hemoptysis C-ANCA Treatment: Steroids, cyclophosphamide
Goodpasture's syndrome	Lung and kidney involvement Hemoptysis and glomerulonephritis	Linear anti-GBM deposits Treatment: Steroids plus plasma exchange
Alport's syndrome	Boys 5–15 years old Asymptomatic hematuria plus nerve deafness plus eye disorder	EM: GBM splitting Treatment: Possible recurrence after transplant
IgA (Berger's) nephropathy	Adolescent male with respiratory or GI infection	IF: Mesangial IgA deposits Increased IgA Treatment: Steroids

Nephrotic Syndrome

Proteinuria > 3.5 g/day, edema, hypoalbuminemia, hypercholesterolemia, foamy urine; see Table 18-4.
Predisposes to hypercoagulable state
Tests: Measure 24-hour urine protein
Key: Fat casts in urine
Treatment (All): Steroids
Other Causes of Nephrotic Syndrome: DM, amyloidosis, lupus, and drugs

TABLE 18-4 Nephrotic Syndrome

Minimal change disease	More common in children	LM and C3—Normal EM—Fusion of epithelial foot processes
Focal segmental glomerulosclerosis (FSGS)	More common in HIV and IV drug users	Biopsy—Sclerotic capillary tufts
Membranous nephropathy	Common in Caucasian adults Associated with syphilis, malaria, HBV	"Spike and dome" IgG and C3
Membranoproliferative nephropathy (MGPN)	Can be a nephritic syndrome	Train-track Type I—Subendothelial deposits Type II—C3 and nephritic factor Type III—Decreased C3

RENAL AMYLOIDOSIS

Patients with chronic inflammatory disease or MM
Congo red stain, apple green birefringence

LUPUS NEPHRITIS

Severity of renal disease directly determines overall prognosis
Subendothelial immune complex deposition

DIABETIC NEPHROPATHY

Increased mesangial matrix
Two forms:
1. Diffuse hyalinization
2. Nodular glomerulosclerosis—Kimmelstiel-Wilson lesions (key)

ACE inhibitors may slow progression.
Diabetes can also cause autonomic neuropathy and detrusor weakness, which leads to overflow incontinence—postvoid urine is high.
FF = (P hydrostatic vessel + P oncotic blood) – (P oncotic vessel + P hydrostatic blood)

RENAL FAILURE

For a representation of renal failure, see Figure 18-3.

FIGURE 18-3 Renal Failure

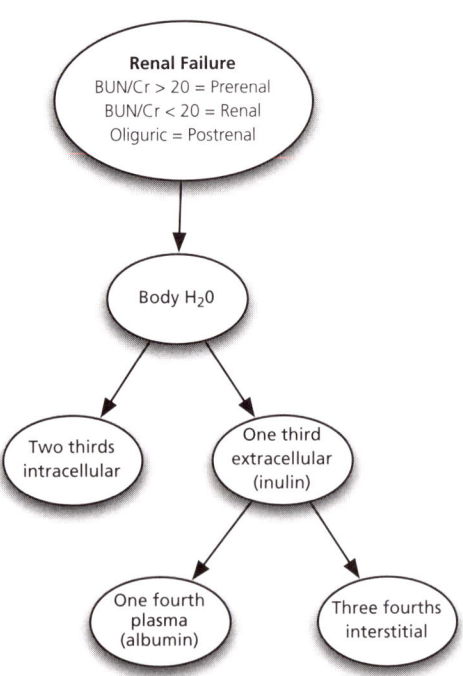

Acute Renal Failure
Progressive rise in BUN/Cr caused by abrupt decrease in GFR
Overall Tests: UA, U/S rules out postrenal; FENa > 3%—renal
For the three types of acute renal failure, see Figure 18-4.

FIGURE 18-4 Three Types of Acute Renal Failure

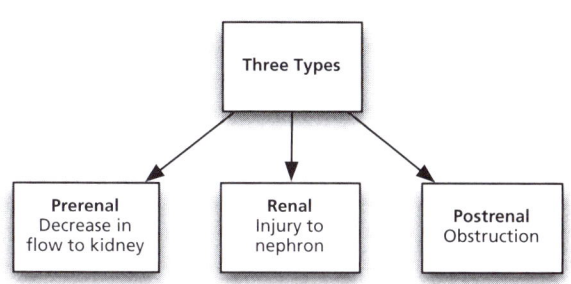

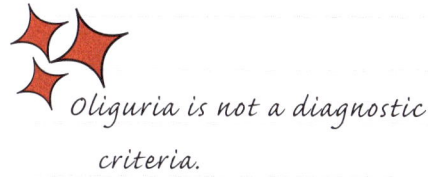

Oliguria is not a diagnostic criteria.

PRERENAL
Hypovolemia!
Cause: Dehydration/hemorrhage, heart failure, sepsis, renal artery stenosis
Keys to Diagnosis:
Prerenal—FENa = (UNa/PNa) / (UCr/PCr)
BUN/Cr—20:1 Urine Na < 20, FeNa < 1%
Treatment: IV fluids, blood

RENAL
Most common type is acute tubular necrosis.
Key to Diagnosis: BUN/Cr 10:1

Myoglobinuria/Rhabdomyolysis
Muscle breakdown interferes with filtration.
Cause: Strenuous exercise, burn, trauma, neuroleptic malignant syndrome, seizure; any condition that will leave you lying on the floor for a prolonged time
Diagnostic: Increased CPK, dark urine
Treatment: Hydration and alkalinize urine

Toxins/Meds
Cyclosporine, aminoglycosides, methicillin
NSAIDs cause papillary necrosis by inhibiting PGs that vasodilate efferent arterioles
IV Contrast: Contraindicated in DM and renal patients (if you must use it, *hydrate*!)—order nuclear scan instead.

Acute Tubular Necrosis (ATN)
Cause: Contrast, aminoglycosides (gentamycin)
Key to Diagnosis: FENa plus excretion > 3%; UA—granular epithelial casts

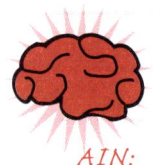

AIN:

"SNAPPeR"

Sulfa, **N**SAIDs, **A**llopurinol,

    Penicillin, **P**henytoin,

    Rifampin

Acute Interstitial Nephritis (AIN)
Caused by drugs
Presentation: Fever, rash, plus renal problems
Diagnostic Tests: High eosinophils, UA—waxy casts

Glomerulonephritis
Kid with strep throat 1–3 weeks earlier
Key to Diagnosis: RBC casts in urine, LM—lumpy
    bumpy

POSTRENAL
Cause: Obstruction distal to kidney
Nephrolithiasis: Must be bilateral in order to cause a
    significant rise in BUN/Cr
Ovarian CA: Older female with bilateral
    hydronephrosis and pelvic mass
Bladder tumor
BPH: (MC) Man over 55 with BPH symptoms
Diagnostic Tests: U/S, IVP
Treatment: Catheterize

Chronic Renal Failure
Same causes as ARF but prolonged
Common Causes: DM, HTN, PCKD
K+ and H+ buildup, uremic pericarditis, bleeding, CNS
    manifestations
Anemia due to lack of erythropoietin
Metabolic acidosis due to impaired renal excretion
Treatment: Dialysis, H_2O-soluble vitamins, Ca+
    carbonate, erythropoietin
See Table 18-5 for urine sediment clues.

Indications for Dialysis:

Hyperkalemia with

    arrhythmia

Uremic encephalopathy

Metabolic acidosis pH < 7.25

TABLE 18-5 Urine Sediment Clues

Waxy casts	AIN
Granular/epithelial casts	ATN
RBC casts	GN
Fat casts	Nephrotic syndrome
WBCs, eosinophils	AIN
WBC casts	Pyelonephritis
Hyaline casts	Can be normal
Leukocyte esterase/+ nitrites	UTI

CHAPTER 19 SURGERY

You should be able to easily earn points from the surgery questions on the test after studying this chapter. Recognizing postoperative causes of fever and ABCs of trauma management are very high yield. Any emergency/trauma situation will be heavily tested on the exam. If it is a situation in which you must diagnose and act quickly to save the patient's life, know how to recognize the diagnosis and the order of steps in evaluation and treatment.

TRAUMA MANAGEMENT

A: Airway
First and foremost, protect the patient's airway! If the blood isn't oxygenated, then it doesn't even matter if the heart is beating.

If the patient can communicate with you, then the airway is adequate. Give supplemental oxygen.

If patient is not communicating, *intubate*. When in doubt, always *intubate*.

B: Breathing
After securing the airway, check to see if the patient is breathing spontaneously. If not, *intubate*.

C: Circulation
With all trauma patients, start two large-bore IV catheters. If patient appears hypovolemic (pale, weak pulse, tachycardic) administer blood and IV fluids. Ringer's solution is almost always used unless patient has renal impairment.

D: Disability
Check neurologic function of patient. Assess GCS; see Table 19-1.

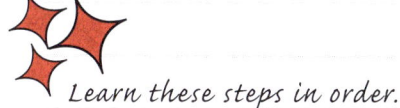

Learn these steps in order.

TABLE 19-1 Glascow Coma Scale (Total 15)

Eye Opening	Motor Response	Verbal Response
Spontaneous 4	Obey 6	Oriented 5
To verbal	Localization 5	Confused 4
commands 3	Flexion 4	Inappropriate 3
To pain 2	Abdominal flexion 3	Incomprehensible
None 1	Extension 2	sounds 2
	None 1	None 1

GCS ≥ 14 Minor head injury

GCS ≥ 9 ≤ 13 Moderate head injury

GCS ≤ 8 Severe head injury

This will help you remember the causes of post-op fever:

Water—UTI

Wind—atelectasis

Walk—DVT

Wound—infection

Weird Drugs—fever caused by drugs and anesthesia

This will help you remember: HG MADE

Just think of these lists and rule things out to reach the correct response.

POSTOPERATIVE FEVER

Need to know the mnemonic and time frame.

Fever 101–102° F
Day 1: Atelectasis
Day 3: UTI
Day 5: Thrombophlebitis
Day 7: Infection
Day 10–15: Deep abscess

PELVIC THROMBOPHLEBITIS
Persistent, spiking, postpartum fever
Treatment: Heparin

INTRA-ABDOMNIAL ABSCESS
Daily fever spikes

Fever 104–105° F
Immediately after instrumentation: bacteremia
Immediately after anesthesia: malignant hyperthermia

POST-OP DISORIENTATION AND COMA

Hypoxia: This is very common; *check blood gas* first!
Glucose: Especially in diabetics
Medication: Very common cause
Ammonia: Commonly seen in cirrhotic patients
DTs: Around post-op day 2 in alcoholics
Electrolytes: Both hypo- and hypernatremia care culprits

POST-OP CHEST PAIN

Pulmonary embolism (PE): 5–7 days
Myocardial infarction (MI): 1–2 days

OBSTRUCTION IN POST-OP PERIOD

Consider adhesions or paralytic ileus
Diagnostic Test: Barium tag

CHEST TRAUMA

For signs and symptoms of chest trauma, see Figure 19-1.

FIGURE 19-1 Chest Trauma

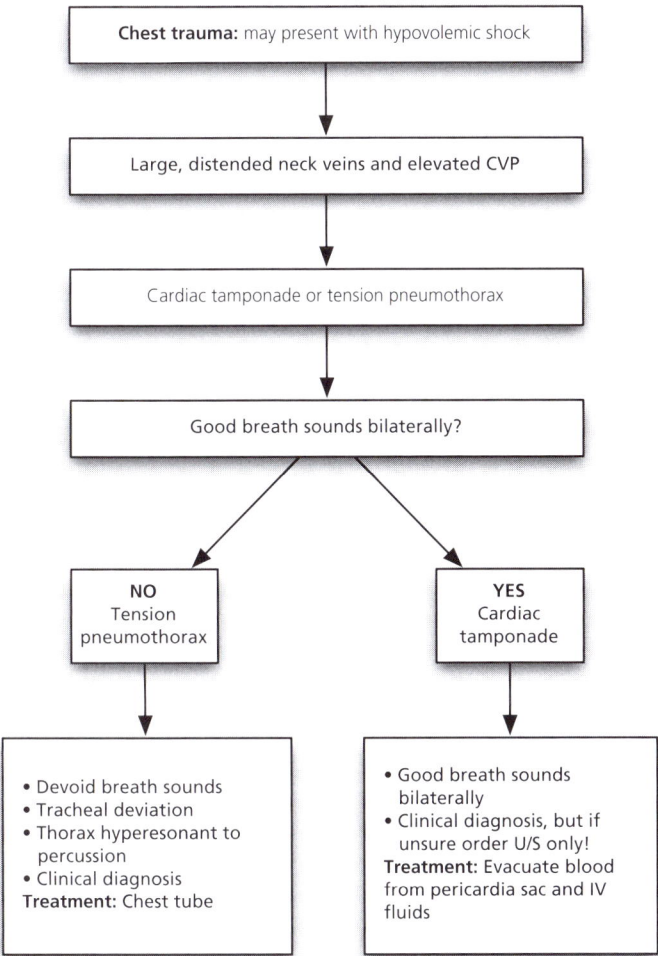

Pnueomothorax is hyperresonant to percussion and may
not present with hypovolemia. If patient is *stable* but
short of breath, you can order chest X-ray to confirm
diagnosis before treatment with chest tube.

Pnuemothorax is *hyperresonant* to percussion and
hemothorax is *dull* to percussion.

Hemothorax: Treat with chest tube to prevent empyema;
the bleeding will stop on its own.

  If chest tube yields a large amount of blood (> 600cc's),
  the bleed is from a systemic vessel. In this instance
  chest tube is not enough, treatment is thoracotomy.

Deceleration injuries to chest, consider myocardial
contusion or aortic rupture; see Figure 19-2.

If patient has broken ribs that are impairing breathing due
to pain, administer local nerve block.

If contusion of lung is suspected, be careful of fluid overload and monitor lung function with ABG.

FIGURE 19-2 Deceleration Injury to Chest

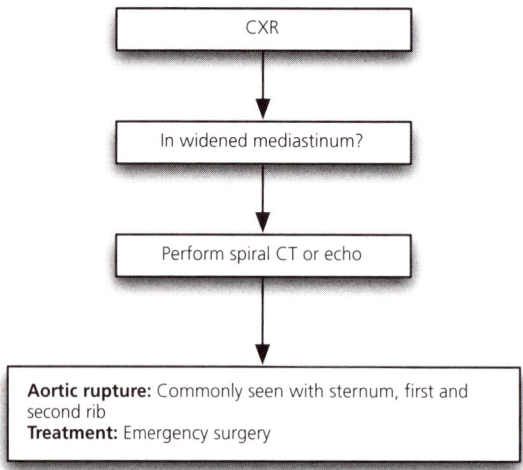

Myocardial contusion is also caused by deceleration injury. If suspected, order chest X-ray and ECG. If ECG is positive, manage like an MI.

PELVIC TRAUMA

Males with pelvic fracture and blood at penile meatus = urethral injury

Tests: Retrograde urethrogram; *do not attempt to pass foley.*

If retrograde urethrogram is negative, pass foley, perform cystogram, and look at postvoid films.

ACUTE ABDOMINAL TRAUMA

If patient is bleeding, treatment is emergency laparotomy; if unsure whether or not patient is bleeding and in ER, perform peritoneal lavage.

If patient is stable and bleeding or if patient is unconscious and bleeding status is unknown, CT with oral and IV contrast.

ACCIDENTAL AMPUTATION

Wrap amputated part in gauze moistened with sterile saline. Place in a plastic bag on bed of ice and go immediately to ER.

OBSTRUCTION

Pain will have sudden onset and *patient will move around in pain.*

Small Bowel Obstruction
Hyperactive bowel sounds, abdominal distension, bilious vomiting
Diagnostic Test: Abdo X-ray shows stepladder appearance or many air fluid levels.
In adults—adhesions (with history of prior surgery).
In children—intussusception, incarcerated hernia.
Treatment: NPO, NG tube, IV fluids, and observation
   If no improvement in 24 hours or fever and leukocytes develop, **surgery**.

Large Bowel Obstruction
Abdominal pain, distension, constipation, and feculent vomiting
In adults—diverticulitis, volvulus (can be decompressed with endoscope), colon CA
In children—Hirschsprung's disease
Sigmoid volvulus: Treat with barium enema
Paralytic ileus: Treat with bethenachol

Diverticulitis
Old patient with LLQ pain
Diagnostic Test: CT scan will confirm
Treatment: NPO, IV fluids, antibiotics
   If several prior episodes, consider surgical intervention.

ABDOMINAL PERFORATIONS

Sudden onset abdominal pain and *patient will lie still*
Diagnostic Tests: Rule out other causes of pain, upright abdominal X-ray, and laparotomy

Pain in Abdominal Quadrants
LUQ: Splenic Rupture
LLQ: Diverticulitis
RLQ: Appendicitis
RUQ: Cholecystitis

In general intestinal obstruction: Adhesions (with history of prior surgery); hernia (no history of surgery)

Obstruction?→U/S

Any older patient with abdominal symptoms, always screen for colon CA!

Abdominal perforations:
Atrial fibrillation + ascites = Mesenteric embolis
Elderly patient + ascites = Sigmoid volvulus or mesenteric ischemia
Chronic ascites = Primary peritonitis

UPPER GI BLEED

For diagnosis of an upper GI bleed, see Figure 19-3.

FIGURE 19-3 Upper GI Bleed

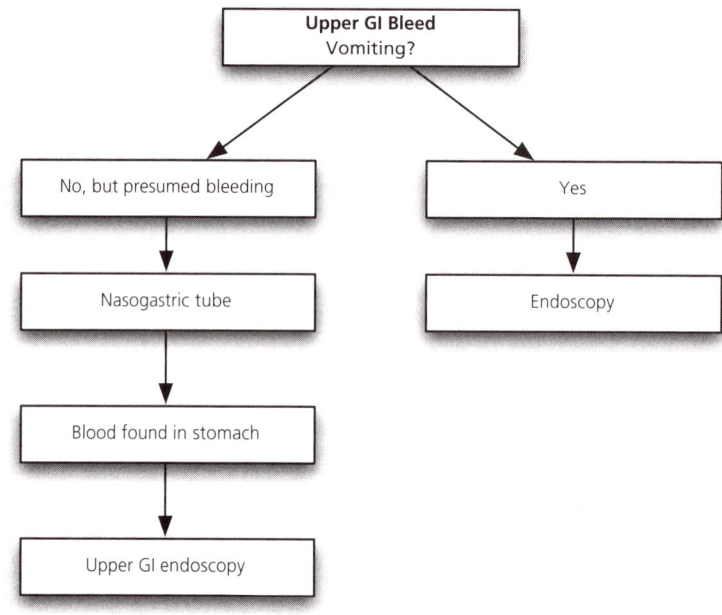

LOWER GI BLEED

More than 2cc per minute, order angiogram.
Less than 0.5cc per minute, order tagged red cell study.

MESENTERIC ISCHEMIA

Bloody diarrhea plus abdominal pain that cannot be
controlled with opioids
Also characterized by long history of abdominal pain after
eating
"Angina of the intestines"

ANGIODYSPLASIA

Colonoscopy reveals "cherry red spots"
Diagnostic Test: Labeled erythrocyte scintigraphy

Predominantly adenocarcinoma
Left side colon presentation: Blood coating stool and change in bowel habits
Right side colon presentation: Anemia
Diagnostic Test: Colonoscopy and biopsy barium shows "apple core" lesion
Treatment: Hemicolectomy and blood transfusion

APPENDICITIS

Presentation: *RLQ pain and anorexia*, nausea and vomiting
Positive Rovsing's sign
Diagnostic Test: U/S or CT scan to confirm but primarily a clinical diagnosis
Treatment: Appendectomy

PANCREATITIS

Patient with history of gallstones or alcohol abuse with epigastric pain that radiates to back
Diagnostic Test: Serum amylase and lipase, CT scan
Treatment: NPO, NG tube, IV fluids, meperidine
Complications: Pseudocyst

SPLENIC RUPTURE

Commonly seen in patients with EBV infection or after blunt abdominal trauma
Positive Kerr's sign
Counsel all patients with EBV to avoid contact sports
Treatment: Splenectomy

BLEEDING ULCER

Patients with history of peptic ulcer plus *no* history of gallstones or alcoholism
Diagnostic Test: Abdominal X-ray shows air under diaphragm
Treatment: Surgical correction

GALLBLADDER DISEASE

Cholangitis
Presentation: *Jaundice*, RUQ pain, fever
History of gallstones

Cholecystitis
RUQ pain, fat, 40, fertile, fever
History of gallstones
Positive Murphy's sign

Diagnostic Test for Cholangitis and Cholecystitis: U/S
Treatment for Both: Cholecystectomy

CAROTID STENOSIS

Presentation: Amaurosis fugax (occlusion of ophthalmic
    artery = ipsilateral blindness), TIA, carotid bruit heard
Diagnostic Test: U/S or duplex scan
Treatment:
    Stenosis < 70% = daily aspirin
    Stenosis > 70% = CEA if patient is stable (best long-term
    prognosis)

ABDOMINAL AORTIC ANEURYSM

Classic presentation is pulsatile mass in abdomen.
Diagnostic Test: Verify size with U/S or CT scan.
May have associated peripheral artery aneurysm.
Treatment: 6 cm or larger—elective surgery; less than
    4cm—check in 2 years; tender on palpation—immediate
    surgery

INTERMITTENT CLAUDICATION

Exacerbated by exercise
Alleviated by rest
Plus associated symptoms of decreased blood flow
    (decreased temp, weak pulse, cyanosis)
Diagnosis: Doppler (if pressure gradient is present, order
    arteriogram)
Treatment: *Must* quit smoking
If disease interferes with work or lifestyle—
    revascularization
Palpable pulsatile mass with bruit and history of
    penetrating trauma—a/v fistula

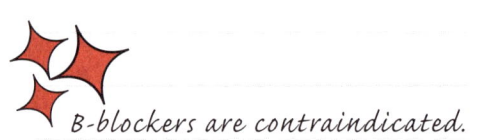
B-blockers are contraindicated.

ULCERS

Venous Ulcer: Medial aspect of leg
Arterial Insufficiency (peripheral vascular disease): Lateral
    aspect of leg plus well circumscribed

Obstructed Lymphatics: Leathery with serous discharge plus whole leg swollen

Varicose Veins: May present with nonpitting edema, medial leg ulcer with brown discoloration of the ankles

    Superficial Thrombophlebitis: Localized pain in superficial leg veins

    Treatment: NSAIDs

HERNIA

Indirect Hernia: Goes *in*to scrotum (most common hernia)

Direct Hernia: Medial to epigastric vessels

Femoral Hernia: More common in females and carries increased risk of strangulation

Treatment for All: Surgery

Complications: Incarcerated hernia is most common cause of small bowel obstruction in patients without history of surgery.

NECK

Zone 1: Neck base

Zone 2: 2 cm above clavicle to mandible angle

Zone 3: Base of skull to mandible angle

Surgical intervention is needed with penetrating trauma to neck plus coughing/spitting up blood, deteriorating vital signs, expanding hematoma.

GSW to Neck:

    Gunshot wound zone 1: Arteriogram

    Gunshot wound zone 2: Exploratory surgery

    Gunshot wound zone 3: Arteriography, esophagogram

Blunt Trauma to Neck: AP lateral, C-spine films, and odontoid views

    If inconclusive, order CT scan.

NEUROSURGERY

Skull

INCREASED INTRACRANIAL PRESSURE (ICP)

There are many causes; just know diagnosis and treatment.

Presentation: Headache, nausea, and vomiting; papilledema; bilateral fixed and dilated pupils

Treatment: Intubate and reverse Trendelenberg

Any signs of increased ICP = contraindication spinal tap; get CT first

Hyperventilate after intubation, this will decrease pCO_2 causing cerebral vasoconstriction = decrease in ICP.

May also use diuretics (mannitol).

If your question stem makes you suspect intracranial bleed of any kind (mention of uncontrolled hypertension, head trauma, alcoholic with possible head trauma), order CT without contrast. Blood will show up white on CT making it easy to recognize.

BASILAR SKULL FRACTURE

CSF from nose or ears, postauricular ecchymosis, periorbital ecchymosis

EPIDURAL HEMATOMA

Usually caused by blow to side of head involving temporal bone causing bleeding from middle ménage artery

Biconvex shaped

Presentation: Head trauma followed by *lucid interval* and then loss of consciousness

Around half present with ipsilateral blown pupil, which is a sign of increased ICP; therefore spinal tap is contraindicated because it may cause uncal herniation.

Diagnostic Test: CT without contrast

Treatment: Craniotomy and decompression

SUBDURAL HEMATOMA

Caused by head trauma that leads to bleeding of bridging veins in cortex and dural sinus

Crescent shaped

Presentation: Classic scenario is *"alcoholic who bumps head"* and presents 1–2 weeks later with neurologic deterioration. Patient may present up to 2 months after insult.

Diagnostic Test: CT without contrast

Treatment: Surgical evacuation

SUBARACHNOID HEMORRHAGE

Caused by trauma or ruptured berry aneurysm causing blood flow between arachnoid and pia mater

Presentation: *"Worst headache of my life"* is the key phrase; patient may also have positive Kernig's and Brudzinski's sign.

Diagnostic Test: CT without contrast (best choice)

Spinal tap is not recommended but reveals grossly bloody CSF.

Cerebral angiogram can locate the defect for surgical intervention.

Treatment: Anticonvulsants and close observation

INTRACEREBRAL HEMORRHAGE

Common causes are hypertension and a/v malformations that cause bleeding in parenchyma.

Bleeding in basal ganglia is commonly associated with hypertension.

Presentation: Contralateral hemisensory deficits and hemiplegia

Diagnostic Test: CT without contrast

Treatment: If possible, surgery

DIFFUSE AXONAL INJURY

Occurs only in severe trauma

Diagnostic Test: CT without contrast will show small punctate hemorrhages and blurring of gray/white mater interface

Treatment: If hematoma is present—surgery; otherwise prevent increase in ICP

Spine

SYRINGOMYELIA

May be caused by cranial malformations or trauma

Cervical or thoracic central cavitation of spinal cord

Presentation: "Cape distribution" loss of pain and temperature sense below lesion

Diagnostic Test: MRI

Treatment: Shunt via surgery

ANTERIOR CORD SYNDROME

Caused by "burst" fracture of vertebral bodies

Loss of pain, temperature, and motor below lesion with preservation of vibratory and position sense

(GENERAL) SPINAL CORD TRAUMA

Look for signs of spinal shock

Hypotension, loss of motor and reflexes

Diagnostic Test: X-rays of affected areas

Treatment: High-dose steroids immediately

Any spinal cord injury— give high-dose steroids immediately, even before test results are back.

CENTRAL CORD SYNDROME

Caused by forced hyperextension of neck via rear-end collision (contra coup); lower extremities normal with paralysis and burning pain in upper extremities

Diagnostic Test: MRI
Treatment: High-dose steroids immediately

SUBACUTE SPINAL CORD COMPRESSION

Usually caused by METS, abscess, or hematoma
Local spinal pain and deficits below lesion
Diagnostic Test: CT or MRI but *give steroids first*
Treatment: High-dose steroids immediately

BROWN-SEQUARD SYNDROME (HEMISECTION)

Clean-cut injury
Contralateral loss of pain sensation distal to injury, ipsilateral paralysis and loss of proprioception

ORTHOPEDICS

See Chapter 14, Table 14-5, "Congenital Hip Diseases and Treatment."
Osgood-Schlatter: Physically active 10- to 15-year-old with *bilateral* knee pain and swelling of tibial tubercle
Scoliosis: Prepubescent girl with lateral curve of back

Fractures

Fractures That Are Badly Displaced: Open reduction and internal fixation
Fractures That Are *Not* Badly Displaced: External manipulation and closed reduction
Diagnostic Tests for All Fractures: Two X-ray views; perform neurological and vascular exams above and below fracture site.

Compartment Syndrome

Caused by prolonged ischemia followed by reperfusion (fracture, burn, or crush injury), commonly seen in forearm and lower leg
Presentation: *Severe* pain with *passive* extension, cyanosis, numbness, paralysis, *elevated* compartment pressure
Treatment: *Immediate* fasciotomy!
Complication: Muscle necrosis and nerve damage

Most common cause of pathologic fracture: Osteoporosis

Pain in anatomic snuffbox: Scaphoid bone fracture

Fracture with highest mortality: Pelvic

Lumbar Disc Herniation

Low back pain caused by herniation of L5–S1 disc (weak plantar flexors, sciatic nerve pain on straight leg raise) or L4–L5 disc (weak foot extensors, pain in groin/hip)

Peak age of onset around 45 years old

Discogenic pain sensed before neurologic pain

Diagnostic Test: CT/MRI

Conservative Treatment: Bed rest; if does not resolve, surgery (diskectomy)

Pain must get worse with cough, sneeze, or strain.

Flaccid rectal sphincter and distended bladder = cauda equina syndrome and requires immediate surgery

Knee Injury

Instablility, pain, and effusion of joint; commonly seen in athletes

Commonly described as "joint popping," "locking up," or loss of full range of motion

Lachman's Test: Knee flexed 90 degrees, push tibia anterior and posterior—assesses ACL and PCL (PCL injuries—check for vascular injury)

Valgus Stress Test: Knee bent 30 degrees, hold knee and abduct ankle—assesses MCL

Varus Stress Test: Knee bent 30 degrees, hold knee and adduct ankle—assesses LCL

Diagnostic Test: MRI

Treatment: Conservative (minor) or surgery (severe)

Osteomyelitis

Most Common Cause: *Staph aureus*

IV drug users and immunocompromised: Gram-negative organisms

Sickle cell anemia: Salmonella

Diagnostic Test: Joint aspiration, Gram stain, culture, and sensitivity

ACUTE HEMATOGENOUS OSTEOMYELITIS

Toddler with febrile illness followed by pain at specific point on bone and refusal to move it

Diagnostic Test: Bone scan (X-ray is useless)

Treatment: Antibiotics (outpatient vs inpatient depends on severity)

Septic Arthritis

Most Common Cause: *Staph aureus*

Sexually active: *Nesseria gonorrhea*

Diagnostic Test: Same as osteomyelitis

Never use steroid drops on eyes; they increase risk of glaucoma and cataracts.

EENT (EYES, EARS, NOSE, THROAT)

Ophthalmology

For neonatal conjunctivitis, see Chapter 14, Table 14-6.

STRABISMUS
Normal until 3 months; if persists—patch good eye

GLAUCOMA
Caused by increased intraocular pressure (IOP)

Most commonly seen in African Americans, older than 40, with family history

90% Are Open Angle: *No* acute attacks

> Characterized by increased IOP and visual field loss
>
> Optic nerve changes = increased cup to disc ratio
>
> **Treatment:** B-blockers, PGs, acetozolamide, pilocarpine

Closed Angle: Acute attacks

Characterized by sudden loss of vision, fixed mid-dilated pupil

Treatment: Pilocarpine drops, oral glycerin, acetozolamide

CENTRAL RETINAL ARTERY OCCLUSION
Sudden, painless, unilateral blindness

Characterized by cherry-red spot on fovea

Treatment: Thrombolytics and high-flow oxygen to decrease IOP

Watch for signs of:

> Temporal arteritis (if present, start high-dose steroids immediately)

Polymyalgia rheumatica

CENTRAL RETINAL VEIN OCCLUSION
Rapid, painless vision loss

Usually seen in elderly

Treatment: Laser photocoagulation

RETINAL DETACHMENT
"Curtain coming down in front of eyes"

Characterized by floaters and flashes of light

OPTIC NEURITIS

Decreased visual acuity and changes in color perception

Blurred disc margins

Commonly associated with *multiple sclerosis* and ethambutol

MACULAR DEGENERATION

Characterized by drusen (white/yellow deposits below retinal pigment epithelium)

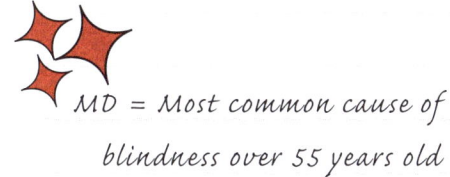

MD = Most common cause of blindness over 55 years old

CATARACTS

Absent "red reflex" in elderly (if in neonate think ToRCHeS)

Slow vision loss

Can be unilateral or bilateral

Affects *lens*

Treatment: Surgery

BILATERAL SUDDEN VISION LOSS

UV Light Exposure: Painful, red, tearing eyes with decreased vision

Seen with tanning bed use, snow skiing, welding

Methanol poisoning

DIABETIC EYE CHANGES

Vitreous (dot-blot) hemorrhage, neovascularization

Treatment: Laser photocoagulation

HYPERTENSIVE EYE CHANGES

Cotton wool spots, copper wiring, a/v nicking

GLASSES

Presbyopia

Decrease in visual acuity caused by normal aging process

"Reading glasses" common in older adults

Myopia (Nearsighted)

Light entering eye falls in front of retina; therefore you must move closer to see properly.

Treatment: Convex lens

Hyperopia (Farsighted)

Light entering eye falls behind retina; therefore you must move further away to see properly.

Treatment: Concave lens

HORDOLEUM
Painful red lump near lid margin, commonly caused by *staph aureus*

CHALIZION
Painless hard lump away from lid margin
Treatment for Both Hordoleum and Chalizion: Warm compress

ORBITAL AND PREORBITAL CELLULITIS
Both include swollen lids, pain, and fever.
If eye movement is impaired, it is orbital cellulitis.
Treatment: Antibiotics (orbital typically requires inpatient treatment)

HERPES SIMPLEX KERATITIS
Dendritic keratitis
Appearance commonly referred to as dendritic spine
Steroids contraindicated
Treatment: Topical antivirals

CN PALSIES AND VISUAL FIELD DEFECTS
CN 3: Eye down and out; if pupil is normal the cause is diabetes or hypertension and will resolve on its own in a few weeks.
CN 4: Affected eye cannot look down when looking medially.
CN 6: Affected eye cannot look laterally.
CN 5 and CN 7: Affects blinking = dry eye.

Blown, nonreactive pupil is an emergency! May be caused by aneurysm; therefore order angiogram or MRI stat.

Ear

HEARING LOSS
Drugs: Loop diuretics, aspirin, aminoglycosides
Tumor: Neurofibromatosis type 2 (CN 8 tumor)

Presbyacusis (Sensorineural)
High-frequency hearing loss bilaterally with difficulty in speech discrimination in older patients
Most commonly caused by aging

Otosclerosis
Progressive **conductive** hearing loss with loss of stapedial reflex
Otic bones appear fixed together
Commonly has family history

Most common cause of acquired hearing loss in children is meningitis.

Sudden deafness at any age can be caused by viral illness.

Ménière's Disease
Hearing loss plus vertigo, nausea and vomiting, tinnitus
Treatment: Antihistamines and anticholinergics

Benign Positional Paroxysmal Vertigo
Nystagmus without hearing loss and vertigo with
  certain head positions
Treatment: Supportive

BELL'S PALSY
Possible cause is reactivation of HSV-1.
URTI followed by unilateral facial paralysis and
  hyperacusis (noise seems louder)

EAR INFECTIONS

Otitis Externa
Commonly caused by pseudomonas—"swimmer's ear"
Pain and discharge from ear canal
Pain with movement of tragus or pinna
Treatment: Antibiotic drops; if diabetic or
  immunocompromised, give IV antibiotics

Otitis Media
Commonly caused by *strep pneumo*, *H. flu*, *Moraxella*
Bulging tympanic membrane
Light reflex and landmarks difficult to visualize

Infectious Myringitis
Commonly caused by mycoplasma, *strep pneumo*, virus
Vesicles on tympanic membrane

Nose

NOSEBLEED
Most common cause is nose picking
Recurrent nose bleed in teenage male *non*-nose picker
  = nasopharyngeal angiofibroma

RHINITIS
Clear nasal discharge
Causes are:
> Viral (common cold)—treat with phenylephrine
> Bacterial (*strep pneumo* or staph)—treat with
>   antibiotics if needed
> Allergic (hay fever—eosinophils in mucus and
>   elevated IgE, nasal crease and dark circles
>   under eyes)—treat with antihistamines or
>   desensitization

Always x-ray nasal fracture and look for septal hematoma.

SINUSITIS

Commonly caused by strep, staph, or *H. flu*

Presentation: Headache, sinus tenderness, green/yellow nasal discharge

Diagnostic Tests: X-ray shows opacification; CT for chronic sinusitis

Treatment: 2 weeks antibiotics; 6 weeks antibiotics if chronic

CAVERNOUS SINUS THROMBOSIS

Headache followed by periorbital edema, fever, and ophthalmoplegia

Throat

NECK MASS

Investigate all masses in neck.

Thyroglossal Duct Cyst: Elevates with tongue protrusion, midline at level of hyoid

Cystic Hygroma: "Mushy" at base of neck

Brachial Cleft Cyst: Located at edge of sternocleidomastoid muscle

Management: Elective surgery

TORUS PALATINUS

20-year-old with immobile fleshy mass on hard palate

Treatment: Reassurance

Enlarged Supraclavicular Node: Abdominal cancer

Long-Term Smoker and Drinker with Neck Mass: Squamous cell cancer METS

Young Patient with Many Enlarged Lymph Nodes: Lymphoma

THYROID CANCER

Most commonly found in young male with history of radiation to neck with single, solid, cold nodule

Does not affect thyroid function and grows slowly

Diagnostic Tests: First U/S then FNA

If malignant—surgery

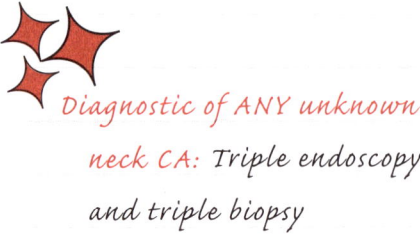

Diagnostic of ANY unknown neck CA: Triple endoscopy and triple biopsy

GENITOURINARY SURGERY

Cryptorchidism
Failure of testes to descend
The more premature, the higher the chance
Treatment: *Wait 1 year*; most will descend on their own.
Orchiopexy is needed after one year of observation.
Orchiopexy is needed to preserve fertility.
Even after surgery **screening for testicular cancer** is
  warranted.
After bringing down the testicle **the chance for testicular
  CA is still increased.**

Testicular Cancer
Cryptorchidism is biggest risk factor.
Presentation: Young male with painless testicular mass
Treatment: Radiation and orchiectomy
Seminoma (germ cell) is most common type.

Hydrocele
Transilluminates
Treatment: Reassurance

Varicocele
No transillumination; may cause pain.
Dilatation of venous plexus.
If symptomatic, treatment is surgery.

Hypospadias
Urethral opening on ventral side
Most common congenital anomaly

Erectile dysfunction
Psychogenic: Presence of nocturnal erections =
  psychological cause
Other causes:
      Vascular
      Medications: B-blockers and SSRIs
      Diabetes
      Renal dialysis
Refer to Chapter 18 for additional information on erectile
  dysfunction.

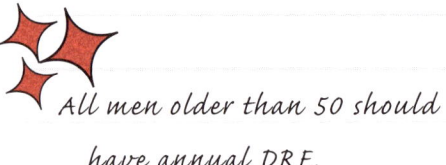

All men older than 50 should have annual DRE.

Testicular Torsion
Presentation: Young male with swollen testes
Prehn's Sign: Testicular elevation = pain same or worse
Treatment: Immediate surgery

Epididymitis
Presentation: Older male with swollen testes and possible urethritis symptoms
Prehn's sign: Testicular elevation = pain decreases
Treatment: Antibiotics

Benign Prostatic Hypertrophy
Normal part of aging
Age of Onset: Around 50 years old
Presentation: Hesitancy, weak stream, incomplete emptying, nocturia
Tests: DRE shows enlarged rubbery prostate; U/A and Cr
Prostate CA DRE = hard lesion or induration
Treatment:
   Mild to moderate disease—terazosin and finasteride
   Moderate to advanced disease—TURP (transurethral resection of prostate)

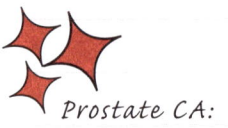

Prostate CA:
Highly elevated PSA is definitive (low elevation may be seen in BPH).

Prostate Cancer
Number 2 cause of cancer death in males
Number 1 cause of cancer in males
Presentation: Urinary retention, weak stream, and back pain, or may be asymptomatic
Diagnostic Tests:
   First: DRE—hard lesion or induration
   Second: U/S-guided transrectal biopsy
   If suspect METS—bone scan and chest X-ray
Treatment: Depends on severity or age; prostatectomy and radiation (follow disease recurrence with PSA)

Bladder Cancer
Risk Factors: *Smoking*, aniline dye, hair dye, infection with schistosomes
Transitional cell carcinoma
Age of Onset: Around 60–70 years old (more common in males)
Presentation: *Gross hematuria*
Tests: U/A, IVP
Diagnostic: Cystoscopy and biopsy
Treatment: Depends on extent of disease

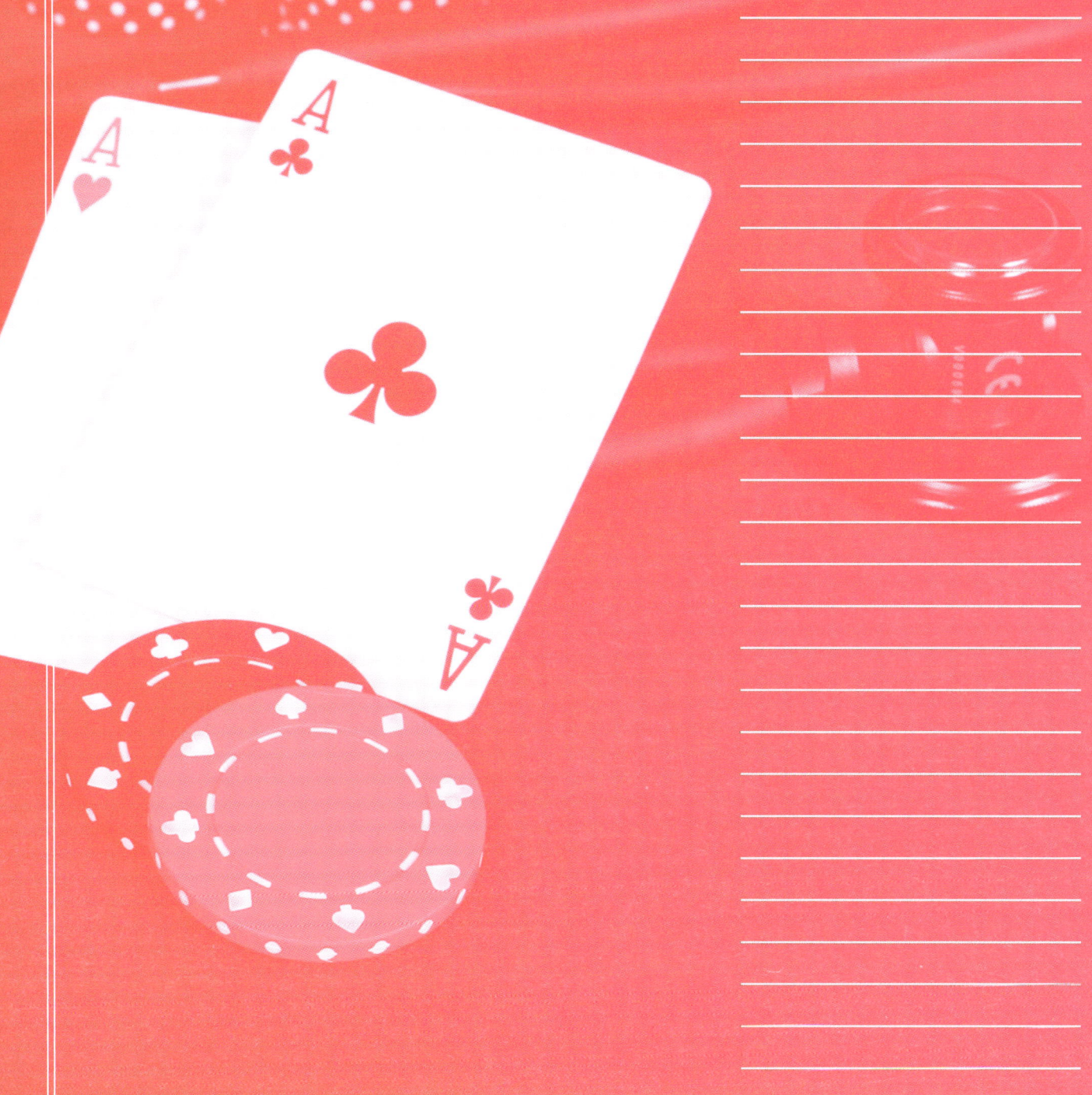

SECTION 2

CLINICAL SKILLS

CHAPTER 20 STEP 2: CLINICAL SKILLS

Included in this chapter are some "pearls of wisdom." I attended a few CS lectures given by the original doctor who created the CS (formerly CSA) exam and its scoring system. During these lectures he revealed some key information you will not find in other books. This section also contains some of my personal experience gained from taking the exam.

COMPONENTS OF THE EXAM

Fees:
> $1200 for IMGs
> $975 for U.S. students

Testing Center Locations: Atlanta, Chicago, Houston, Los Angeles, Philadelphia

Signing Up: Registering for the exam is the same protocol as Step 1 and Step 2 CK. Use the proper Web site, pay the fee, and pick a day.

There are a limited number of testing centers; therefore, it is important to sign up early. I was the first graduating class that was required to take Step 2 CS. It was very difficult to get a date on short notice. I recommend signing up at least 4–5 months in advance. Alternatively, if you do sign up late, it is possible to change your test date without any penalties or charges. There is a calendar online that displays openings at each testing center. If you have to sign up late, make a date and then watch the calendar daily to see what else becomes available. This is really only applicable if you have some time off (for example, during the holidays). It is possible to watch the calendar and take the exam, but you only get a few days' notice.

I signed up late for the test and watched the calendar online. I changed my test date, booked a flight, and flew from New York to Houston and took the exam with only three days' notice. This was only possible because I had already reviewed and practiced for the exam. Learn from my mistake and sign up early!

Passing this exam is required to start residency. Therefore, take it seriously!

Advice for IMGs: Take and pass all of the steps **before** you interview for residency. It is not required, but it will make it easier for you to get the position you want. Also take Step 3 as early as possible.

The test is composed of 11–12 patient encounters lasting 25 minutes each.

- 15 minutes in room with standardized patient
- 10 minutes to complete patient note
- Total test time: 7–8 hours with break and lunch (food is provided by center)

Exam Day: Arrive early on the exam day. Make sure you are well groomed and dressed professionally. Your appearance is taken into consideration via the SP checklist.

Make sure you bring to the testing center:

- Proper paperwork
- Proper ID
- Stethoscope
- *Clean* white coat with *no* logos or emblems
- Clipboards, paper, pens, and all other equipment will be provided for you.

SCORING

1. Communication Skills
English Proficiency (takes the place of the TOEFL):

This should be very simple for native-English-speaking students. If you are an "English as a second language" student, make sure your speech is clear and concise.

- Speaking any language other than English will result in immediate dismissal from the testing center.
- Speaking about cases on the exam, SPs, or anything related is also prohibited.

Standardized Patient Checklist: Completed by SP about your performance

2. Case-Specific Items from History and Physical Checklist:
Asked all the proper questions
Performed the correct physical exam components

The following four components are weighted equally.

Make sure that you do not speak in any language other than English during the exam, even if you see your friend who also speaks that language. There are microphones all over the testing center, even in the bathroom (seriously). If you are heard speaking anything besides English you will not be allowed to continue the exam.

3. Interpersonal Skills
Courteous, professional, established rapport.
Offered proper counseling and appropriate information delivery.
When completing practice cases you will see exactly what the SP's checklist will look like for each scenario; therefore you can practice covering these points.

4. Patient Note
The note can be typed or legibly handwritten. The space provided is small, and you only have 10 minutes. If your handwriting is difficult to read, make sure you type the note. All patient notes are sent to a panel of physicians in Philadelphia to read and score. If they cannot read the note, they cannot award you the points you deserve.

When to Expect Scores
You are supposed to get your scores back in 6–8 weeks. However, be prepared to wait approximately 10–12 weeks for your score regardless of what it says on the USMLE Web site. This is a new test, and they are still refining the scoring process. Consider this extended waiting period as a factor in making deadlines, etc. In addition, some testing centers take longer than others to get your scores back.

Warning: Some of my fellow students took the exam in September and did not get their scores back until December.

STUDY STRATEGIES

This exam does not require as much study time as Step 1 or Step 2 CK, but it does require some preparation. For this exam the amount of prep time you need is directly proportional to the amount of practice you had in clinicals. This is something that you have to gauge for yourself.

I studied for 1 week: 4 days review and 3 days practicing 30 cases with another student.

- Review history taking, physical exam components, tests to order, differential diagnoses, and acceptable abbreviations
- Practice cases (www.usmleworld.com)

If you have limited time, at least practice one scenario from each area (example: 1 abdominal pain case, 1 chest pain case, 1 pediatric case, etc.).

I highly recommend partnering with another student and completing *all* of the usmleworld.com cases. They provide you with every possible scenario. If you have a partner, you can split the cases in half and both have ample practice as "the doctor." This way you learn from each other, and it is much less boring than reading cases on your own.

Review all parts of history taking, physical exam, and completing the patient note.

- Make sure with each scenario you know what questions to ask.
- Familiarize yourself with all physical exam components and make sure that you can do them **quickly**.
- Practice writing the patient note in the standard note form within 10 minutes

TEST PROCEDURE

After a short orientation session, you will be asked to place all of your belongings (including personal pens, paper, etc.) in a room that will be locked for the duration of the test. You also may not leave the testing center building under any circumstances until the day is finished and your test is complete.

All examinees (usually 25 people) line up and are assigned numbers, which are attached to the arms of their white coats. A clipboard, pen, and paper are provided for you. Each person will stand in front of an examination room door. There will be a small window on the door that conceals a sheet of paper.

The paper contains:

- Directions (take history, perform physical exam, discuss findings, or phone consultation, etc.)
- SP's name, age, sex, vitals, chief complaint, and any pertinent history.

All examinees will rotate through all of the exam rooms

HARD-HITTING STRATEGIES

- **Do not look at the paper until time has started**!
- When time begins and you can look at the case, take the time to read it carefully and fully understand what is expected of you **before** entering the room. Take the extra 20–30 seconds to feel confident about what you are about to do. Don't be the person who fails to read the directions, enters the exam room for a phone consultation, and is looking under the exam table for the patient.
- You are provided with scrap paper to take into the encounter with you. You can write whatever you want on this paper because they throw it away and no one will see it. Feel free to write down points that you want to complete **before** you enter the exam room.
- Example: If it is a pediatric case, jot down immunization history, birth history, and feeding history.
- Write down the exam component if necessary (CC, HPI, PMH, PSH, All/Meds, etc.)
- Write down 2–3 differential diagnoses before you enter. This will also help to guide your questions.
- Write down which physical exams you plan to perform. (CV, neuro, and ALWAYS listen to heart and lungs!)
- This may seem silly to you right now, but if you are nervous and enter the exam room with an SP going for the academy award for "problem patient" you will be glad that you wrote down a guideline. The SP's job is to make sure you can perform under any circumstance, therefore he or she will challenge you. Take the 25 seconds to write down a guideline to follow; I guarantee it will save valuable time in the exam room.
- There will be an announcement for 5 minutes remaining. At this point you should already be performing the physical exam. If not, wash your hands while continuing your line of questioning, followed by a transition, and start the PE.
- Remember you want to build in an extra minute or two in case they ask you a challenging question like, "Am I going to die?" Anticipate a challenging question from **each** SP and be prepared.

If you actually are performing a full pulmonary exam, listen to the lungs. To simulate a collapsed lung, the SP will breathe in on one side and only use accessory muscles to raise the chest to simulate pathology on the affected side.

Remember, SPs follow checklists; therefore, if you fail to ask SPs a specific question in a logical order but ask a "go to" question, they will give you the response they learned, and you will get the point.

- When performing the physical exam, be SWIFT. Don't waste time really looking for AV nicking with your ophthalmoscope, trying to assess a murmur, etc.
- Just use the ophthalmoscope; you do not need to see anything. The SP is not really sick! There isn't an attending breathing down your neck waiting for you to report the specific changes of diabetic retinopathy. **By picking up the scope and shining the light in both eyes the SP will grant you points.**
- This is also true with the otoscope—just put it in the SP's ear with a CLEAN tip and you will receive credit.
- For every exam, you must listen to the heart and lungs. This is a very abbreviated exam component. If your stethoscope touches the left side of the chest 3–4 times, that will score you the points for the heart. Score lung points with a few contact points and ask for deep breaths on alternating sides of chest. Use the diaphragm or the bell side of your stethoscope because it doesn't matter to the SP; you will get credit either way. It is one less detail to stress about.

THE "GO TO" QUESTIONS THAT ARE GUARANTEED TO WORK

- Is there anything you would like to add?
- Is there anything else related that you can think of?
- Is there anything else you can remember?

The "go to" questions are great to use when you are washing your hands before the physical exam. They can also be used during the history taking or at the end of the exam. I used them with every SP I had, and they almost always have some additional information.

If you feel you did poorly on a case (typically the first case) do not despair.

Remember, one of the cases is not scored and all cases are averaged to reach your final score. Therefore, if you make a mistake on a case, you can make up for it by shining on your next case.

Props

Watch SPs closely. Occasionally they will have props.

- If they are coughing, offer them a drink of water.
- If they are sneezing, offer them a tissue.
- If the SP has a tissue, ask to see it and check it for sputum and/or blood.
- If the patient has a cane, crutches, or walker, make sure you ask them how long they have been using the device and if it aids mobility.

Questions

- Look for and inquire about tremors or contractures.
- To simulate trauma SPs will wear makeup simulating bruises or other markings. Ask about these areas and handle them expeditiously.
- If you are performing the physical exam and you recall a question you forgot to ask during the history, don't hesitate to ask. This could equal another point.
- Don't attempt to examine the patient over clothes.
- Never feel uncomfortable or embarrassed to ask an SP a question. Sex, drugs, or erectile dysfunction—ask about it! You can't offend them, they're actors!

Alcohol and Tobacco

Always ask if the SP drinks alcohol, how much, and how often. If the SP drinks more than 2–3 drinks per day, ask the CAGE questions.

CAGE

- Have you ever felt the need to **C**ut down on your drinking?
- Have you ever felt **A**nnoyed by criticism of your drinking?
- Do you ever feel **G**uilty about drinking?
- Have you ever needed an "**E**ye opener" in the morning to steady your nerves?

Ask the CAGE questions even if the SP is a sweet little 70-year-old religious woman who looks like your granny. Trust me—you will not offend the professional patient. The CAGE questions are usually on the SP checklist. Include this in your note as a CAGE score; 2/4 CAGE questions.

TOBACCO

Always ask if the SP uses any tobacco products.

If the answer is yes, always ask how much per day and if he or she has considered quitting, and offer counseling. Record smoking as packs per day and number of pack years (for example, 2 packs per day for 26 pack years).

COMPONENTS OF EVERY SP'S CHECKLIST

Wash hands: After taking the history, wash your hands and use a "go to" question before starting the physical exam. It is a good transition and the SP will always add information.

Use the foot rest: Extend the foot rest for any exam that requires the patient to be supine. You will not get points for letting the SP's legs dangle. Always aid the patient in moving on and off the examination table and during any applicable maneuvers.

Do not inflict unnecessary pain on the SP: If the SP shows ANY discomfort, do not perform the maneuver again. If you inflict pain after a warning, you will not receive a point.

Rapport: Smile, act genuinely concerned, and be nice! Even if the SP is acting like a "difficult patient," never lose your cool. Sit at or below patient eye level during the history taking and keep an open relaxed posture.

Act attentive at all times!

EXAMPLE OF INTERPERSONAL CHECKLIST

_____ 1. **Knocked on exam room door before entering**
Do not wait for a response from the knock, enter immediately, establish eye contact, state the patient's name, shake hands, and introduce yourself.

_____ 2. **Made appropriate eye contact**
Start making eye contact from the moment you enter the room and keep it up for the entire encounter.

_____ 3. **Proper introduction of him/herself**
Clearly identify yourself—specify your name and rank (fourth-year medical student, or if you are already a doctor in another country use "Doctor" as your title).

_____ 4. **Used respectful draping**
Always be respectful of the patient! Only expose the area being examined. Don't whip off the patient's entire gown to do an abdominal exam. When you enter the room a sheet will be folded up on a stool. To make sure you don't forget, after the introduction go ahead and place the sheet on the patient's bare legs. This way you are guaranteed a point.

_____ 5. **Remained attentive and expressed genuine concern (2 points)**

_____ 6. **Asked one question at a time**
Use clear, short, easy-to-understand questions. The fewer words the better.

_____ 7. **Phrased open-ended questions**

_____ 8. **Used close-ended questions appropriately**
I consider these questions the "yes or no" style questions. Proper use of these questions usually comes after a transitional statement or introduction of a line of questioning. For example, after telling the patient you would like to ask questions about his or her family history. "In your family, is there a history of diabetes? Thyroid disorders? In the past have you ever had surgery?" etc. If the patient answers yes, you can allow him or her to clarify and fully explain the circumstances.

_____ 9. **Allowed patient to answer without interruption**
If a patient is trying to tell you something, _especially an SP_, listen! Always allow them to finish their train of thought; this automatically makes you seem attentive and concerned.

_____ 10. **Used understandable (nonmedical) language**
Use layperson's language at all times. If you use any medical terminology immediately follow it with an understandable explanation of what you mean. For example, "I think you may have osteomyelitis, which is an infection of the bone."

_____ 11. **Introduced transitional statements**

This allows you to direct the interview. For example, "Now I would like to ask you about your sexual history," or "I would like to learn more about your past medical history."

_____ 12. **Summarized**

Always recap the information the SP gives you. A good time to do this is after completing the history of the presenting complaint.
For example, you could say, "I would like to clarify what we have gone over so far: You are experiencing burning upon urination which began 2 days ago that has progressively gotten worse since onset," etc. "Is this correct?"

_____ 13. **Talked during physical exam**

The last thing you want to hear from an SP is "What are you doing back there?" A good way to start is to always ask permission to begin the physical exam and untie the gown.
Announce that you are going to touch the patient.
"I am going to place the stethoscope on your back so I can listen to your lungs." It is also important to explain to the patient what you are doing and why you are doing it. "I am going to press on your legs for signs of water retention."

_____ 14. **Discussed preliminary findings and impressions**

After the physical exam, explain what you think the diagnosis might be. Explain to the patient that you will have a more definite idea after running some tests and that you would like to see them for a follow-up appointment.

_____ 15. **Discussed tests to order**

Tell the patient what investigations you plan to order and why: "I would like to have a blood test done to check for signs of infection."

_____ 16. **Gave appropriate reassurance**

Always act in accordance with your findings. The patient will ask a "challenging" question. For example, "Am I going to die?" Or "It's cancer; my father had cancer; it must be cancer. Do you think I have cancer?" Be realistic; explain to the patient that you will need to run tests to determine that. Also provide a comforting statement such as, "Let's not think the worst," or "I will be here to help you."

_____ 17. **Asked if there were any questions/concerns**
Always ask patients if they have any questions and take the time to fully answer them. Ask the patients if there is anything else they are concerned about or would like to discuss.

Practice all of these skills and you are guaranteed these points.

ALTERNATIVE ENCOUNTERS

Different encounters have different requirements.

Follow-Up: Some encounters explain that the patient was seen previously and you are required to discuss lab results—and are not required to take a history, perform a physical exam, or write a patient note. This encounter is testing your interpretation, and you will be expected to counsel. A good example of this type of encounter is a young woman with an STD. You would be expected to explain what the results mean, and ask all of the sexual history questions and gyn history questions. Counsel her on how the disease is transmitted and always ask about HIV infection risk factors, exposure, and testing. Explain how infection can be prevented in the future and ask whether or not she would like to bring in her partner for treatment and counseling.

Phone Consultation: Your instructions will tell you to go into the exam room and pick up the phone; you will be connected automatically with the person you need to speak to. For example, the angry, overworked mother with a sick infant. In this scenario take a full pediatric history and explain to the mother that she must bring the child in for you to examine him or her before making a diagnosis or implementing a treatment plan. Do not cave, even if she says she has no legs, no car, and no money for a cab; suggest the bus or tell her you will send an ambulance to pick up her and the child.

Simulators: It is projected that in 2006 that there will be a patient encounter that contains simulators for pelvic and breast exams. As silly as it may seem, follow the directions on the door and act as professionally as possible.

Pediatric Encounters: There are pediatric encounters on the exam, but there is no child SP present. The encounter will be directed through the mother or over the phone.

Do not attempt to perform a rectal, pelvic, or breast exam on a standardized patient. The SPs interact with many examinees each day; I don't think they would appreciate it. They are implementing simulators for those exams. If you have an SP with a chief complaint that warrants a pelvic, breast, or digital rectal exam, write that in the investigation portion of your patient note.

TAKING A FULL MEDICAL HISTORY

Taking a history from an SP is much easier than taking a history from a real patient in reference to questions about prior surgeries, meds, or family history. The SP knows all dates of past surgeries, medications with dosages, and all pertinent family history—QUICKLY. You will not spend time fishing through a grocery bag full of medication that a patient brought or try to figure out the surgical history of a patient with dementia. **The SPs are ready to give you the answer including the generic names of medication.** If real life were only this easy!

General Medical History
Questions to ask all **Standardized Patients:**

- **Name**
- **Age**
- **Address**
- **Occupation**—occupation is listed in social history portion
- **Presenting complaint** (chief complaint): This should be "in the patients own words"; therefore let them fully explain why they are seeking medical attention at this time.
- **History of presenting illness** (for example, pain):
    Onset: When did you first notice it?
    Duration: How long has this been happening?
    Radiation: Does the pain radiate or move anywhere or is it always in the same place?
    Location: Can you point to where you feel the pain with one finger?
    Frequency: How often do you experience it?
    Pain scale: On a scale of 1 to 10, 0 representing no pain and 10 being childbirth/a shard of glass in the eye/a kidney stone, etc., how would you rate your pain?

Character: Would you say your pain is sharp, dull, stabbing, gnawing, etc.?

Exacerbating/alleviating factors: Can you think of anything that makes it better or worse?

Precipitating factors: Can you think of anything that could have brought this on?

Progression: Do you feel it has gotten worse since its onset?

Meds taken: Did you try any pain relievers to ease the pain?

Any other symptoms: Are you experiencing any other problems with this? This is a good way to go into the review of systems

- **Review of Systems (ROS):** Have you experienced any:
  Nausea/vomiting?
  Diarrhea/constipation/change in bowel habits?
  Increased urinary frequency/urgency/change in urinary habits?
  Fever/chills?
  Sore throat/headache?
  Chest pain/shortness of breath/cough?
  Appetite or weight change?
  Dizziness/problems sleeping?
  Any pain *anywhere?*
  Have you traveled anywhere recently?

- **Past medical history:** Ask if they have any coexisting, prior, and childhood illnesses. If so, inquire when they occurred.

- **Surgical history:** Ask if they have ever had surgery before. Or you could say, "Have you ever been hospitalized for any reason before?" This statement can cover a broad range of things.

- **Family history:** Ask about any illnesses in the family, parents, siblings, grandparents, etc., and record which family member was afflicted (maternal grandmother, paternal grandfather, etc.). A good way to phrase it is "Are your parents/siblings still living, and are they healthy?" "Do your parents or siblings have a history of heart disease, cancer, or thyroid disease?" You may also want to mention one or two diseases related to the patient's own history or chief complaint. Ask an African-American patient if there is any sickle cell disease present in the family. You don't need to ask an SP if 20 different specific diseases have afflicted family members. SPs are scripted; they anticipate the

Always try to ask about travel. It can provide valuable clues about the patient's condition.

family history portion of the interview and will offer the information.

- **Allergies:** *Always* inquire whether or not they have any allergies to medications and, if so, what type of reaction they had. Also ask if they suffer from any other type of allergy (food, etc.).
- **Medications:** Always inquire what medications the patient is currently taking—prescription, OTC, and herbal products.
- **Social history:**

  What do you do for a living?

  Who do you live with? or Do you live alone? Married/single/children?

  Do you use any tobacco products? How often? If the patient is a smoker, record number of packs per day and number of pack years.

  Do you drink alcohol? What type of alcohol do you drink? How many units of alcohol per week?

  Do you use any recreational drugs?

  Sexual history—Are you sexually active and with whom?

  What type of contraception do you use?

  If the patient is not married, ask how many sexual partners he or she has had in the last year. Men, women, or both?

  Ever had a sexually transmitted disease? and When was your last HIV test, and what was the result?

  If suspected, ask about erectile dysfunction. For example, dialysis patients almost always suffer from this problem.

  ROS

Special Histories

PEDIATRIC HISTORY

Birth and Delivery History

Was the pregnancy full-term? Were there regular prenatal check-ups?

Number of weeks gestation at delivery?

Was it a complicated pregnancy?

What type of delivery, vaginal or C-section?

Was it a complicated delivery? How long was the delivery?

Any other prior pregnancies and outcome?

Feeding History

Breast or bottle fed? Any problems feeding?

When did the child begin eating solid foods?

What sort of things does he/she regularly eat and how is his/her appetite?

Does the child have any allergies?

Routine Care and Immunization History

Are immunizations up to date?

When was the last pediatric visit? What was the outcome?

Has the child had previous hospitalizations or serious illnesses?

Ask about developmental milestones, height, weight, etc.

OB/GYN HISTORY

Inquire about sexual history if not already asked.

Menstrual Cycle

How old were you when you first had your period?

How many days are in your cycle? Is it regular? Have you noticed any changes in your cycle?

When was the first day of your last menstrual period? Or if applicable ask when menopause started. Any associated symptoms (hot flashes)?

Do you experience any bleeding in between periods?

On average, how many pads/tampons do you use per day?

How would you characterize your flow? Light/normal/ heavy?

OB

Have you ever been pregnant, and what was the outcome? Include number of children and any abortions or miscarriages.

PSYCHIATRIC HISTORY

General

How have you been feeling?

Can you tell me about anything that could have caused you to feel this way?

How long have you felt like this?

Support

Do you have anyone you can talk to?

Daily Routine (interests, activities, eating, sleeping)

What is your normal routine like? Have you noticed any changes?

What kind of interests/activities/hobbies do you have? Any change? Do you still engage in and enjoy these things?

How many hours per night do you sleep? Have you noticed any change in your sleep pattern?

Have you noticed any change in your eating habits? Any weight gain or loss?

Caffeine

How much caffeine do you consume per day?

Concentration/Memory

Have you had any difficulty concentrating or remembering things?

Future

How do you feel about your future/? Do you have any future plans?

Do you think things will get better or worse for you?

Hallucinations/Delusions

Do you hear or see things that other people do not hear or see? How long? What do they say?

Suicide

Do you ever think about killing yourself/ending it all?

Do you have a plan? What is your plan? Do you already have the guns/pills/bridge picked out, etc.?

Do you ever think about harming others?

Abuse

Inquire about any bandages, bruises, or signs of abuse present.

What is it like for you at home?

Do you feel safe at home?

Is there anyone at home who treats you badly? What is your relationship like with the people/person you live with?

Were you harmed or left alone as a child?

Family History

Has anyone in your family experienced similar problems to the ones you are having?

Thyroid Function

Do cold or hot temperatures frequently bother you?

Do you have problems sleeping?

Do you ever get constipated?

Have you noticed any changes in the thickness or texture of your hair?

Has your skin been dry lately?

Seeking Help

Would you be willing to talk with someone who could help you with these problems? I can refer you to some people who can help you.

HOW TO HANDLE PROBLEM PATIENTS AND DIFFICULT QUESTIONS

In handling these patients it is best to *always* start with

1. "Yes, Mr./Ms. _____, I understand" etc.
2. Follow first statement with: Corresponding "answer" below.

Financial Worrier

Patient: "Doctor, I don't have insurance, and I do not think that I can afford this."

Answer: "Don't worry about that. I can have someone from social services speak with you. They offer options to help you with these issues. Your health is priceless, so let's focus on that right now."

Addict

Patient: "I know I should stop smoking, but I just don't think that I can."

Answer: "I know that it is difficult to stop smoking, but I am concerned about your health. There are many treatment options to help you stop smoking. I can help you find one that is right for you. Would you be willing to try to quit?"

Angry

Patient: "I have been waiting here for 2 hours, and no one has even been by to check on me. I know you people think your time is more important than mine and that I should just wait my turn!"

Answer: "I know that your time is very important, and I deeply apologize for your long wait time. It has been unusually busy today. I am here to help you, and you have my undivided attention."

Hypothyroidism is commonly misdiagnosed as depression.

It is a good idea to use the patient's name. It shows that you are paying attention, and it helps to establish a relationship with the patient. The SP will interpret this as establishing rapport.

Pain

Patient: "Doctor, I am in a lot of pain. I think I need something right now to take the edge off."

Answer: "I think it is best if we wait until I have a better idea of what is causing the pain, and I can prescribe the medication that will work best for you. I understand that it is uncomfortable, but it will only be a few minutes."

Work Worrier

Patient: "My boss does not like for me to miss work; I hope I don't get fired."

Answer: "After the examination I will write you a doctor's note for the proper amount of time you will need to take off."

Genius

Patient: "No, Doctor, you are wrong. You must be mistaken; it is _____."

Answer: "Thank you; I appreciate you telling me that. Let me explain and/or clarify."

Resistant

Patient: "I never get sick. There is nothing wrong with me; I am fine. I only came in so my husband/wife would get off my back."

Answer: "What does your wife/husband think is wrong with you? I am here to help you." Or, "Since we are both here, I should take a history and perform a quick physical."

Rude

Patient: "I don't want a woman/foreign doctor."

Answer: "I know it is uncomfortable coming to the doctor, but I am here to help you. I am very well trained, and I will make sure that you will get the best care possible."

Death Worrier

Patient: "Do I have cancer?" Or "Is it serious?"

Answer: "There are a few possibilities for the diagnosis. It could be _____ or _____. To be sure, I need to run some tests. I will study the results and we can meet again to review everything. At that time we can discuss which treatment option would be best for you."

Renal
Have you ever had any:
Difficulty urinating?
Pain/discomfort when urinating?
Blood in urine?
Increased frequency/urgency?
Men:
> Has your urinary stream changed?
> Have you had any reduction of urinary stream?
> Dribbling?
> Hesitancy/difficulty initiating urination?

Neurologic
Have you ever experienced any:
Dizzy spells/felt light-headed?
Fainting spells/seizures?
Numbness/tingling?
Weakness/paralysis?

Gastrointestinal
Have you experienced any:
Heartburn?
Difficulty swallowing?
Abdominal pain?
Vomiting? How many times? Does it contain blood?
Have you noticed a change in your bowel habits? Caliber?
    Color?
Have you noticed a change in your appetite/weight?

Breast
Do you regularly do breast self-exams?
Have you noticed any lumps in your breast?
Have you ever had any pain in your breast?
Have noticed any changes in the skin on your breast?
Have you ever noticed any nipple discharge? What color
    was it? Was it on both sides?

Respiratory
Have you had any:
Difficult breathing?
SOB?
Have you had a cough? Is it productive? If so, what color is
    it?
Chest pain?

Musculoskeletal
Do you ever experience any:
Pain in your joints?
Swelling/redness?
Stiffness?
Do these symptoms ever limit your daily activities?

Cardiovascular
Do you ever have chest pain?
Palpitations?
Shortness of breath?
How many pillows do you sleep on?
Are your ankles ever swollen?

PHYSICAL EXAM

Perform a very abbreviated CV and respiratory exam on *all* patients. Quickly listen to heart and lungs. If you put your stethoscope on the patient's chest a few times, you will receive credit.

GI

Inspect the abdomen for scars, striae, veins, size, shape, color, symmetry, and any visible movement (pulsatile or peristalsis).
Auscultate (one area).
Palpate starting away from area of pain.
Light palpation of all four quadrants.
Deep palpation of all four quadrants (look for masses or tender areas).
Look for fluid wave and shifting dullness.
Assess the tip of spleen.
Percuss the borders of liver and spleen.
Ballot kidneys.
CVA tenderness—have patient sit up and pound on flank.
If appendicitis is a possibility—Rovsing's sign.
Psoas sign.
Obturator sign.
Rebound tenderness: ask the patient if he or she feels any pain.
Cholecystitis: Murphy's sign.
Boas's sign.
If DRE is warranted, put it in the investigations portion of the patient note.

CV

Look for sign of cyanosis, clubbing, etc.
Check pulses.
Assess BP.
Check for edema (pedal).
Recline patient (45 degrees).
Inspect JVP.
Look for any scars and inspect precordium.
Palpate the cardiac areas: aortic, pulmonic, tricuspid, mitral.
Palpate for thrills.
Auscultate all areas with bell and diaphragm; repeat in
    reverse with and bell.
Have patient lie on left side and listen to mitral.
Have patient sit up.
Listen to cardiac areas again.
Have patient lean forward and listen to cardiac base.
Listen to carotid arteries for bruits. Ask patient to hold
    breath while auscultating each side.

Peripheral Vascular System
Examine hair, nails, skin
Compare all four extremities for size, symmetry, and feel
    for temperature
Look for signs of low blood flow (ulcers, lack of hair
    growth, etc.)
Palpate pulses: radial, ulnar, brachial, femoral, popliteal,
    posterior tibial, dorsalis pedis
Allen's test
Burger's test
Trendelenberg test
Pratt's test
Homan's test

RESPIRATORY

Look for presence of cyanosis, finger clubbing, and use of
    accessory muscles.
Inspect nose and throat.
Palpate trachea and look for deviation.
Perform steps on back first; then repeat on anterior.
        Check for deformities and symmetry.
        Test for tactile fremitus (99) (4 areas).
        Percuss symmetrically, alternating right and left starting
            at apex (6 areas).

Auscultate symmetrically alternating right and left (6 areas).

Note breaths sound character, resonance.

Whispered pectoriloquy.

MUSCULOSKELETAL

Inspect and palpate each joint group for redness, swelling, deformity.

Test active range of motion; if active is impaired, check passive range of motion.

Test strength/power.

Test reflexes.

Knee Joint

Bulge/ballotement

McMurray's test: Knee flexed 90 degrees, hold heel with other hand and internally rotate ankle while extending the knee. Repeat using external rotation. Perform all maneuvers bilaterally.

Lachman's test: Knee flexed 90 degrees push tibia anterior and posterior = assesses ACL and PCL (PCL injuries check for vascular injury)

Valgus stress test: Knee bent 30 degrees, hold knee and abduct ankle = assesses MCL

Varus stress test: Knee bent 30 degrees, hold knee and adduct ankle = assesses LCL

Straight Leg Raise

Sciatic nerve compression

Thomas's test

Phalen and Tinel's test: Check for median nerve compression

NEUROLOGICAL

Mini-mental status exam—alert, oriented, concentration, memory

Ask patient about time (current season or today's date) and location (state, town, etc.).

Tell the patient 3 objects, have the patient repeat them, and tell the patient to remember them.

Serial 7's.

Ask the patient to recall the 3 objects.

Cranial Nerves

CN 2, 3, 4, 6: Test visual acuity (Snellen's provided)
Corneal reflex and pupillary reflex (direct and consensual)
Accommodation
"H" test (tests EOM and test convergence)
CN 5: Pain, fine touch, and mastication
CN 7: Smile, close eyes, wrinkle forehead, blow out cheeks
CN 8: Weber, Rinne, and whisper tests
CN 9, 10: Open up and say "ah" to test soft palate movement
CN 11: Assess trapezius and sternocleidomastoid muscles; shrug shoulder against resistance and turn head against resistance.
CN 12: Ask patient to stick out tongue and move it from side to side.

Sensory

Assess crude and fine touch, pain, and vibratory sense.
Proprioception of fingers and toes: have patient close eyes, move toe and ask up or down.
Romberg's test: indicates cerebellar lesion.
Vibration—use tuning fork.

Sensation

2-point discrimination: normal is 4-5 mm.
Point localization: With patients' eyes closed, touch them and then have them identify the point you are touching.
Extinction: Touch the patient on the trunk or legs in one place or in two places simultaneously and then tell the patient to open his or her eyes and point to the location where he or she felt sensation.
Stereognosis: Have patients close their eyes, put a familiar object in their hand, and ask them to identify it.
Graphsthesia: Ask patients to close their eyes and identify the number or letter you will trace with the back of a pen on their palm.

Cerebellum

Ask the patient to:
Walk in a straight line heel to toe.
Walk in a straight line on heels.
Walk in a straight line on toes.
Finger–nose test: Instruct patient to alternate touching the tip of their nose with one finger and then touch your finger, which you are holding up. Then move your finger around and have patient continue the exercise.

Ask patients to take the heel of their left foot, touch their right shin, and move their left heel from knee to shin. Repeat with opposite foot on opposite leg.

Rapid alternating movements: Ask patient to flip hands from back to front.

Motor

Look for fasciculations, tremor, or atrophy.
Palpate muscle groups in limbs for tone.
Test all muscle groups for power.
Check all reflexes.

HEAD, EYES, EARS, NOSE, AND THROAT (HEENT)

Head/Neck

Examine and/or palpate head: size, shape, symmetry, scars, and facial expressions.

Inspect scalp (swelling deformity) and hair (distribution, amount).

Inspect inside of mouth, including all parts and dentition (note hygiene).

Examine and palpate neck: lymph nodes, trachea, thyroid gland, and check tracheal alignment.

Ask patient to swallow and watch thyroid gland movement.

Palpate thyroid and ask patient to swallow.

Ear

Check external ear for signs of inflammation or deformity.

Palpate mastoid process, auricle, tragus. Always ask, "any pain or discomfort?"

Use otoscope and note state of tympanic membrane; perforations, incus, color, malleus. Always place clean tip on otoscope.

Weber test: Place tuning fork on the center of the top of the head. "Do you hear it in both ears?"

Rinne test: Place tuning fork by ear and instruct patient to tell you when he or she does not hear the sound anymore. Then place the base of the tuning fork on bone behind ear and ask, "Do you hear it now?" Perform bilaterally.

Whisper test: While standing to the side of the patient whisper a word and ask the patient to repeat the word you whisper. Perform bilaterally.

Nose

Inspect nostrils for color, discharge, symmetry, deviation.

Palpate maxillary and frontal sinuses.

Eyes

Look at brows and lids for retraction, swelling, ptosis, scars, and alignment.

Note health of conjunctiva, lacrimal punctae, sac, and anterior chamber.

Visual acuity: Instruct patient to cover one eye and read the smallest line he or she can see on Snellen eye chart.

Peripheral vision: Wiggle fingers in imaginary sphere on sides of head. Ask patient to look forward and raise their hand on the appropriate corresponding side when he or she first notices your fingers.

"H" test: Ask the patient not to move his or her head and to follow your fingers with their eyes only. After performing the "H," this is a good time to test convergence by moving your finger from midpoint of H to tip of the patient's nose.

Assess pupillary reflex and reactivity (direct/consensual) and shape. Dim lights and use the ophthalmoscope's white beam (check on back of hand first) to shine on lateral side of left and right eye. Note constriction of pupils in both eyes.

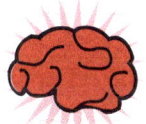

Right, right, right

Use ophthalmascope to look into the patient's eyes; remember, use your right hand and right eye to look into patient's right eye.

Before you begin, ask the patient to focus on a spot on the wall and try not to blink.

WHEN TO DO EXAMS

Neuro	Dizziness/balance problems
	LOC
	Seizure
	Visual disturbance
	Psych
	Weakness/paralysis/parasthesia
	Headache
HEENT	Trauma
	Headache
	Sinus pain
	Eye: eye pain, ocular disturbance
	Ear: ear pain, hearing loss, tinnitus
	Nose: rhinorrhea, epistaxis
	Throat: sore throat, dysphagia, jaw pain
CV	Chest pain
	SOB
	Palpitations
	Pedal edema
	LOC
Respiratory	Chest pain
	SOB
	Wheezing
	URI symptoms: cough
Abdominal	Change in bowel habits
	Abdominal pain
	Pelvic pain, or any OB-GYN complaint
	Urinary symptoms, increased frequency, urgency, etc.
	Jaundice
	Rectal bleeding
Musculoskeletal	Decreased ROM
	Joint pain, stiffness, swelling
	Extremity pain
	Muscle pain, weakness

SAMPLE PATIENT NOTE

Patient Note

History:

Physical Exam:

Differential Diagnosis

1.

2.

3.

4.

5.

Diagnostic Work-up

1.

2.

3.

4.

5.

HOW TO WRITE A PATIENT NOTE

General

Typed or handwritten, it is your choice. You can practice both styles and see which one works best for you.

Do not write fake findings in your patient note. If the SP has pneumonia, don't record the findings as what you **should** hear. Record what you actually hear or see from the simulation the SP provides. The doctors that score the note are interested in the organization and legibility of the note; therefore, don't fabricate answers.

Concentrate on making your note complete, with all components, normal findings, proper documentation, and abbreviations. This is what the note is scored on.

It doesn't matter if you get some of the differential diagnoses or tests wrong; just try to be in the "ballpark."

The patient note should be neat, organized, and cohesive.

Specific

CC: A statement explaining why the patient is seeking medical attention. This should start with age and gender; for example: 36 yo male c/o.

HPI: Document all of the details surrounding the chief complaint. Example: Location, radiation, exacerbating/alleviating factors, onset, duration, pain scale, etc.

PMH: Past illnesses, hospitalizations, surgeries, with dates.

Allergies/Medications: List allergy and reaction; food, meds, etc. Note any meds the patient is currently taking prescription, OTC, or herbal.

FH: Cancer, DM, thyroid disease, etc. Designate which family member.

SH: Single, married, children, job, smoking, ETOH, recreational drugs, sex; OBGYN, psych, if relevant.

PE: Start with a statement about vital signs. Point out anything abnormal and write WNL for the rest.

Write a general statement about the patient's general appearance. For example, patient is comfortable, in no apparent distress, or agitated and in apparent distress.

Make an organized list of important positives and negatives. List the positives that may rule out certain diagnoses. Example: If a patient c/o chest pain, but lungs are clear, write, "Lungs clear to auscultation bilaterally."

Diagnostic Work-up: List in order you would want them performed.

When ordering tests (U/S, X-ray, MRI, or CT) don't forget to put which area. For example, Chest X-ray, Head CT.

Include breast, rectal, and pelvic exams in this section.

Never order referrals, consults, or hospital admit.

Differential Diagnoses: List possibilities in order from most likely to least likely.

Do not leave this space completely blank.

Try to come up with at least three differentials.

Do not include long shot diagnoses to fill in the extra space.

NORMAL EXAM DOCUMENTATION

Abdominal: No scars, striae, skin abnormalities on inspection.

Bowel sounds present.

Abdomen is soft, nontender, with no masses detected on palpation.

No CVA or rebound tenderness.

CV: Pulses 2+ bilaterally BP _____ HR _____.

No palpable heaves or JVD detected; PMI not displaced, no evidence of pedal edema.

Normal S1/S2 with regular rhythm.

No rubs, gallops, or murmurs heard.

HEENT: Head atraumatic, normocephalic.

Eyes: EOM intact, normal convergence, PERRLA; no evidence of papilledema or fundoscopic abnormalities.

Ears: Clear tympanic membranes and canals WNL bilaterally.

Nose: No discharge, normal nasal turbinates.

Throat: No tonsillar exudates or enlargement.

Neck: Supple, no lymphadenopathy, no thyroid enlargement

Mouth: Good dentition, no lesions

Respiratory: Lung fields clear to auscultation and percussion bilaterally

No rhales, rubs, or wheezes

No signs of cyanosis

Tactile fremitus WNL

Neuro: Alert and oriented x 3, good concentration

CN II–XII intact

DTR 2+ bilaterally

All groups 5 out of 5 muscle strength

Negative Babinski, Tinel, Kernig, Brudzinski

Negative Romberg

Sensation intact bilaterally

Musculoskeletal: Normal ROM
No signs of joint pain, swelling, or crepitus
Anterior and posterior drawer sign WNL
Muscle strength 5 out of 5 all groups
DTR 2+ bilaterally
Mini mental status: Patient appears well groomed
Alert and oriented x 3
Recent and remote memory are intact
Serial 7's shows good attention and concentration
Affect consistent with mood, judgment intact

COMMON TESTS TO ORDER

Abdominal:
LFTs
Pancreatic amylase, lipase
CT abdomen
B-HCG
Pelvic exam
Endoscopy
Sigmoidoscopy
Colonoscopy
ERCP
DRE
Occult blood test
U/S (specify quadrant)
Abdominal X-ray
CBC with diff
BUN, Cr, U/A, urine culture

CV:
CBC with differential
ECG
CXR
Carotid Doppler
CK-MB, troponin
Electrolytes

Musculoskeletal:
X-ray
CT
MRI
Nerve conduction studies
Biopsy muscle
ESR
EMG

CBC with differential
Joint aspirate, culture, crystals
_____ antibody

Pulmonary:
Pulse oximetry
ABG
CBC with differential
CXR
CT scan chest
Spirometry
Sputum studies (culture, gram stain, India ink)
PPD

Psych:
TSH/T3/T4
CT brain
MRI brain
Electrolytes
Toxicology screen
Urine catecholamines
HIV

ABBREVIATIONS

Here are the acceptable abbreviations used in the patient note portion of the clinical skills exam. In the real world, hundreds of abbreviations are widely used in the practice of medicine.

CAUTION: The following are the **only** patient note abbreviations acceptable on the CS exam. Make sure you practice writing your patient note using only abbreviations from this list.

–	negative
+	positive
ABG	arterial blood gas
AIDS	autoimmune deficiency syndrome
b	black
B-HCG	beta human chorionic gonadotropin
BP	blood pressure
BUN	blood urea nitrogen
C	Celsius
CBC	complete blood count
CHF	congestive heart failure
Cig	cigarette
CK level	creatine kinase
Cm	centimeters
COPD	chronic obstructive pulmonary disease
CT	computerized tomography
CV	cardiovascular
CVA	cerebral vascular accident
CXR	chest X-ray
DM	diabetes mellitus
DRE	digital rectal exam
DTR	deep tendon reflexes
ECG	electrocardiogram
ENT	ear, nose, throat
EOM	extraocular muscles
ESR	erythrocyte sedimentation rate
ETOH	alcohol
Ext	extremity
F	Fahrenheit
f	female
FH	family history
G_p_	gravida para

GI	gastrointestinal
GU	genitourinary
HEENT	head, eyes, ears, nose, throat
HgA1C	hemoglobin A1C
HIV	human immunodeficiency virus
HR	heart rate
Hr	hour
HTN	hypertension
hx	history
JVD	jugular venous distension
JVP	jugular venous pressure
Kg	kilograms
L	left
Lbs	pounds
LFT	liver function tests
LP	lumbar puncture
M	male
Mg	milligram
MI	myocardial infarction
Min	minute
MRI	magnetic resonance imaging
MVA	motor vehicle accident
Neuro	neurology
NIDDM	non-insulin-dependent diabetes mellitus
NKA	no known allergy
NKDA	no known drug allergy
NSAID	nonsteroidal anti-inflammatory drugs
NSR	normal sinus rhythm
OBGYN	obstetrics/gynecology
Oz	ounces
PERRLA	pupils equal, reactive to light accommodation
PT	prothrombin time
PTT	partial prothrombin time
R	right
RBC	red blood cell
ROM	range of motion
TIA	transient ischemic attack
TRH	thyroid releasing hormone
TSH	thyroid stimulating hormone
U/A	urinalysis
URI	upper respiratory infection
Vs	vital signs
w	white
WBC	white blood cell
WNL	within normal limits
yo	year old

ABBREVIATIONS IN THIS BOOK AND BEYOND

–	negative
+	positive
5HIAA	serotonin
AAA	abdominal aortic aneurysm
Ab or ab	antibody
Abd	abdomen
ABG	arterial blood gas
Ach	acetylcholine
ACTH	adrenocorticotropic hormone
AD	autosomal dominant
ADH	antidiuretic hormone
AF	atrial fibrillation
AFP	alpha fetoprotein
AIDS	autoimmune deficiency syndrome
AIN	acute interstitial nephritis
Alk phos	alkaline phosphatase
ALL	acute lymphoblastic leukemia
ALS	amyotrophic lateral sclerosis
AML	acute myelogenous leukemia
ANA	antinuclear antibody
ANCA	antineutrophil cytoplasmic antibody
ANOVA	analysis of variance
AR	autosomal recessive
ARDS	adult respiratory distress syndrome
ASA	aspirin
ATN	acute tubular necrosis
AV	atrioventricular
AVM	arteriovenous malformation
AVP	arteriovenous pressure
b	black
B-HCG	beta human chorionic gonadotropin
B/L	bilaterally
BM	bone marrow
BP	blood pressure
BT	bleeding time
BUN	blood urea nitrogen
Bx	biopsy
C	Celsius
CA	cancer or carcinoma
Ca+	calcium
CABG	coronary artery bypass graft
CAD	coronary artery disease
CBC	complete blood count
CEA	carcinoembryonic antigen

CHF	congestive heart failure
Cig	cigarette
CIS	carcinoma in situ
CK	creatine kinase
CK level	creatine kinase level
Cm	centimeters
CMV	cytomegalovirus
CN	cranial nerve
CNS	central nervous system
Coag	coagulation
COPD	chronic obstructive pulmonary disease
COX	cyclo-oxygenase
CPAP	continuous positive airway pressure
CS	clinical skills
CSF	cerebrospinal fluid
C-spine	cervical spine
CT	computerized tomography
CV	cardiovascular
CVA	cerebral vascular accident
CVP	central venous pressure
CXR	chest X-ray
DES	diethylstilbestrol
DHEA	dehydroepiandrosterone
DI	diabetes insipidus
DIC	disseminated intravascular coagulation
DKA	diabetic ketoacidosis
DM	diabetes mellitus
DM II	diabetes mellitus type 2
DMD	Duchenne muscular dystrophy
DNI	do not intubate
DNR	do not resuscitate
DOC	drug of choice
DRE	digital rectal exam
DTR	deep tendon reflexes
DTs	delerium tremens
DUB	dysfunctional uterine bleeding
DVT	deep venous thrombosis
EBV	Epstein-Barr virus
ECG	electrocardiogram
ECHO	echocardiogram
ECT	electroconvulsive therapy
ED	erectile dysfunction
EDD	estimated date of delivery
EEG	electroencephalogram
EF	ejection fraction

ELISA	enzyme-linked immunosorbent assay
EM	electron microscopy
EMG	electromyogram
ENT	ear, nose, throat
EOM	extraocular muscles
EPS	extrapyramidal symptoms
ERC	endoscopic retrograde cholangiopancreatography
ESR	erythrocyte sedimentation rate
ETOH	alcohol
Ext	extremity
F	Fahrenheit
f	female
FENa	fractional excretion of sodium
FEV	forced expiratory volume
FF	filtration fraction
FFP	fresh frozen plasma
FH	family history
FHR	fetal heart rate
FNA	fine needle aspiration
FSH	follicle-stimulating hormone
FTA-ABS	fluorescent treponemal antibody-absorbed
FVC	forced vital capacity
G_p_	gravida para
G6PD	glucose-6-phosphatase deficiency
GAD	generalized anxiety disorder
GBM	glomerular basement membrane
GCS	Glasgow coma scale
GDM	gestational diabetes disorder
GERD	gastroesophageal reflux disease
GFR	glomerular filtration rate
GI	gastrointestinal
GnRH	gonadotropin releasing hormone
GTT	glucose tolerance test
GU	genitourinary
HA	headache
HAV	hepatitis A virus
Hb	hemoglobin
Hb F	hemoglobin fetal
Hb S	hemoglobin sickle
HbA1c	hemoglobin A 1c
HCG	human chorionic gonadotropin
HCT	hematocrit
HDL	high-density lipoproteins
HEENT	head, eyes, ears, nose, throat

Hep B or HBV	hepatitis B virus
HgA1C	hemoglobin A1C
HHV-6	human herpes virus
HIDA	hepato-iminodiacetic acid (scan)
HIV	human immunodeficiency virus
HLA	human leukocyte antigen
HMG CoA	hydroxymethylglutaryl-coenzyme A
HPI	history of presenting illness
HPV	human papilloma virus
HR	heart rate
Hr	hour
HRT	hormone replacement therapy
HSV	herpes simplex virus
HTN	hypertension
HUS	hemolytic uremic syndrome
hx	history
IBD	inflammatory bowel disease
IBS	irritable bowel syndrome
ICP	intracranial pressure
IF	immunofluorescence
IFN	interferon
Ig	immunoglobulin
IHSS	idiopathic hypertrophic subaortic stenosis
IMA	inferior mesenteric artery
INH	isoniazid
INR	international normalized ratio
IOP	intraocular pressure
IPV	inactivated polio vaccine
ITP	idiopathic thrombocytopenic purpura
IUD	intrauterine device
IUGR	intrauterine growth retardation
IVDU	intravenous drug user
IVP	intravenous pyelogram
JVD	jugular venous distension
JVP	jugular venous pressure
Kg	kilograms
KOH	potassium hydroxide
KUB	kidney, ureter, bladder
L	left
LA	left atrium
LAD	left anterior descending coronary artery
LAP	left atrial pressure
LBBB	left bundle branch block
LBP	lower back pain
Lbs	pounds

LFT	liver function tests
LMP	last menstrual period
LP	lumbar puncture
LUQ	left upper quadrant
LV	left ventricle
LVH	left ventricular hypertrophy
M	male
MAOI	monoamine oxidase inhibitor
MAP	mean arterial pressure
MC	most common
MCA	middle cerebral artery
MCL	medial collateral ligament
MCP	metacarpophalangeal (joint)
MCV	mean corpuscular volume
MDD	major depressive disorder
METS	metastases
Mg	milligram
MI	myocardial infarction
Min	minute
MM	multiple myeloma
MMR	measles, mumps, rubella vaccine
MRA	magnetic resonance angiography
MRI	magnetic resonance imaging
MS	multiple sclerosis
MSAFP	maternal serum alpha fetoprotein
MVA	motor vehicle accident
N and V	nausea and vomiting
NCV	nerve conduction velocity
NE	norepinephrine
Neuro	neurology
NF	neurofibromatosis
NG	nasogastric (tube)
NICU	neonatal intensive care unit
NIDDM	non-insulin-dependent diabetes mellitus
NKA	no known allergy
NKDA	no known drug allergy
NPO	nil by mouth
NSAID	nonsteroidal anti-inflammatory drugs
NSCLC	non-small cell lung cancer
NSR	normal sinus rhythm
NST	nonstress test
O_2	oxygen
OBGYN	obstetrics/gynecology
OCD	obsessive compulsive disorder
OD	overdose

OPV	oral polio vaccine
OTC	over the counter
Oz	ounces
p	pressure
PAS	periodic acid schiff
PCKD	polycystic kidney disease
PCOS	polycystic ovarian syndrome
PCP	phencyclidine hydrochloride or pneumocystis carinii pneumonia
PCR	polymerase chain reaction
PDA	patent ductus arteriosus
PE	pulmonary embolus
PEEP	positive end-expiratory pressure
PERRLA	pupils equal, reactive to light accommodation
PFT	pulmonary function test
PG	prostaglandin
PID	pelvic inflammatory disease
PIP	proximal interphalangeal (joint)
PMN	polymorphonuclear lymphocytes
PND	paroxysmal nocturnal dyspnea
PPD	purified protein derivative (tuberculosis)
PPI	protein pump inhibitor
PPV	positive predictive value
PROM	premature rupture of membranes
PSA	prostate-specific antigen
PT	prothrombin time
PTH	parathyroid hormone
PTT	partial prothrombin time
PUD	peptic ulcer disease
PVC	premature ventricular contraction
R	right
RA	right atrium
RBC	red blood cell
RDS	respiratory distress syndrome
REM	rapid eye movement
RF	rheumatoid factor, risk factor, or rheumatic fever
RLQ	right lower quadrant
ROM	range of motion
RPR	rapid plasma reagent
RSV	respiratory syncytial virus
RTA	renal tubular acidosis
RTI	respiratory tract infection
RV	right ventricle

S&S	signs and symptoms
SAH	subarachnoid hemorrhage
SCA	sickle cell anemia
SCC	squamous cell carcinoma
SCFE	slipped capitol femoral epiphysis
SIADH	syndrome of inappropriate antidiuretic hormone
SIDS	sudden infant death syndrome
SLE	systemic lupus erythematosus
SOB	shortness of breath
SP	standardized patient
SSRI	serotonin specific reuptake inhibitor
STD	sexually transmitted disease
TA	temporal arteritis
TAH-BSO	total abdominal hysterectomy—bilateral salpingopherectomy
TB	tuberculosis
TBG	thyroxine binding globulin
TCA	tricyclic antidepressant
TE or TE fistula	transesophageal
TIA	transient ischemic attack
TIBC	total iron binding capacity
TIPS	transjugular intrahepatic portosystemic shunt
TMP-SMX	trimethoprim sulfa
TOF	tetralogy of fallot
TORCH	toxoplasmosis, other, rubella, cytomegalovirus, herpes
tPA	tissue plasminogen factor
TRH	thyroid releasing hormone
Trt	treatment
TSH	thyroid stimulating hormone
TSS	toxic shock syndrome
TSST	toxic shock syndrome toxin
TTP	thrombotic thrombocytopenia purpura
TURP	transurethral prostatectomy
Tyr	tyrosine
U/A or UA	urinalysis
U/S	ultrasound
UC	ulcerative colitis
UMN	upper motor neuron
URI	upper respiratory infection
UTI	urinary tract infection
V/Q	ventilation perfusion ratio
VC	vital capacity

VDRL	venereal disease research laboratory
VF	ventricular fibrillation
VS	vital signs
vs	versus
VSD	ventricular septal defect
VT or V tach	ventricular tachycardia
vWF	von Willebrand factor
VZV	varicella zoster virus
w	white
WBC	white blood cell
WNL	within normal limits
WPW	Wolff-Parkinson-White syndrome
XR	x-linked recessive
yo	year old

INDEX